CANADIAN BACK INSTITUTE

THE CBI METHOD TO

End Your Back and Neck Pain

Hamilton Hall, M.D.
Illustrated by M. B. Mackay

SEAL BOOKS
McClelland-Bantam, Inc.
Toronto

This book is not intended to replace the services of a physician. Any application of the recommendations set forth in these pages is at the reader's discretion and sole risk.

The CBI Method to End Your Back and Neck Pain
A Seal Books original publication/September 1996

For information, address: Seal Books

ISBN: 0-770-42712-X

Seal Books are published in Canada by McClelland-Bantam, Inc. Its trademark, consisting of the words "Seal Books" and the portrayal of a seal, is the property of McClelland-Bantam, Inc., 105 Bond Street, Toronto, Ontario M5B 1Y3, Canada. This trademark has been duly registered in the Trademark Office of Canada. The trademark consisting of the words "Bantam Books" and the portrayal of a rooster is the property of and is used with the consent of Bantam Books, 1540 Broadway, New York, New York 10036, USA. This trademark has been duly registered in the Trademark Office of Canada and elsewhere.

Cover design by Melody Cassen
Cover photography courtesy Comstock
Text design by Heidy Lawrance Associates
Printed and bound in Canada

CONTENTS

ACKNOWLEDGMENTS

Thank you to all the Canadian Back Institute staff in clinics across Canada who have worked to develop and refine the techniques described in this book.

Special thanks to Tony Melles, Senior Clinician and Executive Director of CBI for his help in preparing this manuscript and, in a much larger sense, for helping to create the method itself.

INTRODUCTION

This book can help you eliminate neck and back pain. Its goal is to provide more than necessary information and long-term strategies. Its aim is to give you the ability to stop your pain right now.

The strategies are the result of over 20 years' experience with the Canadian Back Institute (CBI). The exercise routines described reflect those employed by more than 30,000 patients a year to abolish acute episodes of neck and low back pain. Long-term control is fundamental but immediate pain relief is more urgent. This book teaches you how to achieve it.

Exercise is important although the word often implies long hours in a gym or fitness club. The exercises in this book should more properly be termed "pain control maneuvers". Like conventional exercise they require that you make an effort, but unlike those sessions in your sweat-suit, the physical effort is limited and the results can be instantaneous. Incorporated into your everyday activities, the techniques you learn here can make the difference between seemingly endless bouts of pain and mere minutes of discomfort.

The first stage of the CBI program, focused on symptom control, addresses not only exercise but posture as well. A few minutes of movement cannot compensate for hours in the wrong position. You may be surprised to learn that a specific activity, a sudden twist or heavy lift, usually has less to do with neck or back pain than does sustained poor posture. Sitting awkwardly when reading this book may be enough to trigger an attack.

Here is a program with exercises that you can manage. It offers a simple approach that will help you move and sit more comfortably. The CBI method can help to end your neck and back pain … today!

YOUR SPINE

Your spine extends from the base of your skull to the top of your pelvis. Although its structure changes slightly along its length, the basic elements remain the same. The bones of your back are called vertebrae. The front of each bone, the body, is shaped like a drum lying on its side. Attached to the back of the drum is a ring of bone surrounding the spinal cord and emerging nerves. Projecting from the back of the ring are four bony knobs creating two pairs of joints which link each vertebrae to the one above and the one below. Also protruding from the ring are bony spines that anchor the muscles.

Separating the vertebral bodies are discs. These fibrous, jelly-filled shock absorbers allow the spine to stay flexible while supporting both your body weight and the weight of anything you lift. In the neck (the cervical spine) bones become smaller and the discs thinner. The interlocking joints are flat and slope backwards from above down. These smooth plates allow considerable movement but render this

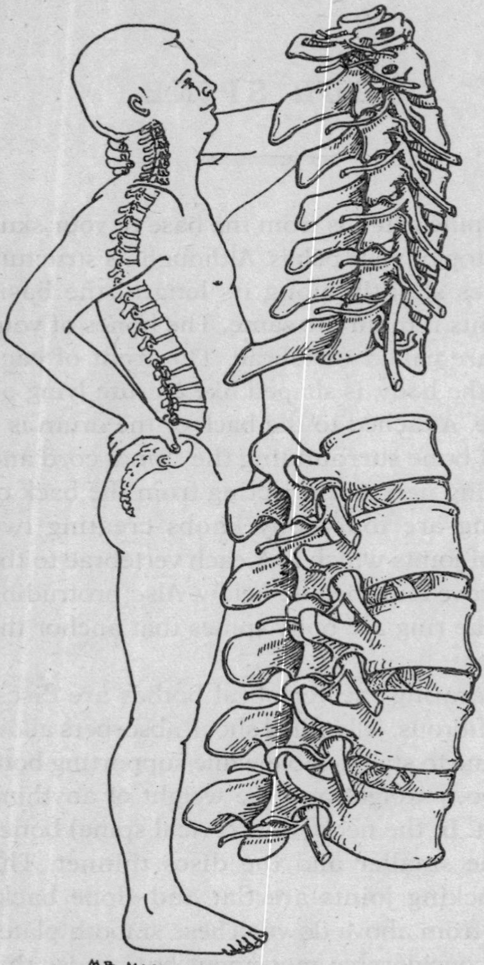
M.B. MACKAY ©

portion of the spine more susceptible to joint irritation.

The low back, or lumbar spine, consists of five large vertebrae. The discs are much thicker and the interlocking joints are shaped like the letter "L". This configuration adds stability but limits movements.

The spinal cord lies within a continuous bony tunnel, the spinal canal, made up of the rings of bone attached to the back of each vertebrae. Branches from the cord exit the canal between adjacent vertebrae and create the nerves that travel throughout the body.

Five nerve roots in the neck come together to fashion all the nerves in the arms. Four roots in the low back coalesce to form the sciatic nerve running down the back of the leg.

In addition to providing a sense of touch and directing muscles to move, nerves convey pain. As it leaves the spine, every nerve root sends

Although the vertebrae in the low back are larger, the cervical and lumbar spine have many similarities. Nearly half the neck movement occurs at the two levels immediately below the skull. Flat, mobile spinal joints further increase the range of cervical movement while angled, interlocking joints reduce movement in the low back. Both areas have strong discs, a tunnel protecting the spinal cord and multiple exit holes for the spinal nerves.

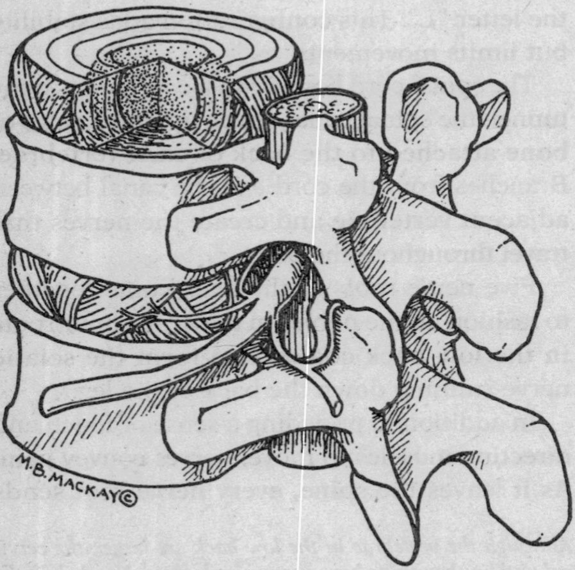
M.B. MACKAY©

pain-reporting fibers to the structures it passes: the disc, the small joints, the ligaments and the muscles. With such a rich nerve supply it is hardly surprising that backs hurt so often and after even trivial insults.

Because the nerves that allow your spine to feel pain provide the same service to your limbs, signals originating from a disc or back joint may be felt down your arm or leg. When discomfort in the spine is felt somewhere else, the process is termed "referred pain". The effect is common and typical of most mechanical back problems. This type of pain must be distinguished from the pain of a pinched nerve, which can also travel into the arms or legs. After a nerve pinch, the pain is accompanied by signs of direct nerve involvement such as the slight decrease in power in a specific group of muscles. Although most back pain sufferers consider the pinched nerve to be a common affliction, actually only one sufferer in ten experiences the problem. Most back pain simply comes from an unwanted load on the spine itself.

A jelly-like center is surrounded by fibrous outer rings that anchor the disc to the vertebral bodies. The local nerve supply insures that the disc, the joints and the covering of the nerve itself are capable of feeling pain.

pain-reporting fibers to the spine: this is passed to the disc, the small joints, the ligaments and the muscles. With such a rich nerve supply it is hardly surprising that backs hurt so often and after even trivial insults.

Because the nerves that allow your spine to feel pain provide the same service to your limbs, signals originating from a disc or back joint may be felt down your arm or leg. When discomfort in the spine is felt somewhere else, the process is termed "referred pain." The effect is common and typical of most mechanical back problems. This type of pain must be distinguished from the pain of a pinched nerve, which can also travel into the arms or legs. After a nerve pinch, the pain is accompanied by signs of direct nerve involvement such as the slight decrease in power in a specific group of muscles. Although most back pain sufferers consider the pinched nerve to be a common affliction, actually only one sufferer in ten experiences the problem. Most back pain simply comes from an unwanted load on the spine itself.

[illegible] nerve itself are incapable of feeling pain.

YOUR PAIN

Patterns One, Two, Three and Four

This program is intended to relieve mechanical pain, the most common type of back and neck complaint. The term "mechanical" indicates that the source of the symptoms is one of the physical components of your spine, the bones, discs or joints. The term also implies that the pain has nothing to do with much rarer but more serious causes such as infection, tumour or generalized disease.

Over 95 percent of back and neck pain is mechanical in nature. This type of pain typically has three characteristics. First, the symptoms are aggravated by particular movements and relieved by other movements or brief periods of immobility. Second, the pain increases while holding certain positions and decreases with a change in posture. Both points make sense when you remember that the source of most back or neck pain is merely irritation of a sore disc, joint or ligament. The situation is similar to suffering a sprained ankle. Walk on it or hold it the wrong way and it hurts: move it carefully or find the correct rest position and it feels better immediately.

The third common characteristic of mechanical back pain is its intermittent nature. The pain commonly comes and goes as the offending structure is alternately loaded and unloaded. That's why your neck and back will continue to hurt as long as you go on doing things that irritate them. Sometimes the elements are so sensitive that even periods of rest or corrective posture will not totally alleviate the pain. Movement and position still produce the expected fluctuations in discomfort but the pain never disappears completely. It becomes constant.

You can't damage your spine with normal activity. Although frequent repetition of the same movement or prolonged maintenance of a normal posture can cause pain, hurt doesn't mean harm. Using your back in the wrong way causes unnecessary pain and getting rid of pain is what this program is all about.

During an acute attack it may be difficult to remember a time when your back or neck didn't hurt. Although pain holds your attention, the diagnosis of mechanical spinal problems concentrates not on the amount of pain but on the particular characteristics of the episode. Mechanical pain should not be associated with accompanying symptoms such as fever, weight loss, skin rashes or persistent problems with other joints. A careful account of the pain itself should allow your attack to be placed into one of four distinct patterns. Allowing for the obvious differences between the neck and low back, the patterns are similar in both areas of the spine.

Pattern One describes pain aggravated by forward bending. In the neck, this means looking down, resting your chin on your chest. In the low back, this means everything from shovelling, raking and vacuuming to making the bed or picking up the groceries. Since most of us tend to slump forward while we sit, sitting increases the pain in both the neck and low back.

Pattern One pain can be constant or intermittent and is felt predominantly along the spine. In the neck, most of the pain is present at the base of the skull, along the tops of the shoulders or between the shoulder blades, and can be associated with a headache that radiates as far as the forehead. In the low back, the pain is primarily in the small of the back below the belt line, across the top of the pelvis, and in the buttocks.

Based on the initial response to a backward movement, there are two types of Pattern One pain. When this movement diminishes the typical pain the patient is termed a "fast responder". Presumably because of the residual flexibility of the spine, appropriate exercises will have a rapid effect. Pattern One pain increased by bending backward as well as by bending forward indicates a "slow responder". The greater loss of spinal mobility makes all movement painful, directs treatment towards posture correction and predicts a prolonged recovery.

Pattern Two pain is always intermittent and never increased by forward bending. It is felt in the same locations as Pattern One but is aggravated by arching backward, for example, by painting the ceiling or flying a kite. The pain is reduced by sitting or bending forward. Episodes appear more suddenly and resolve more rapidly than Pattern One attacks.

Most neck pain is related to a sustained head forward posture and is Pattern One. The brief appearances of Pattern Two are more related to specific movements than to a fixed position.

Pattern One is also the most common pattern in the low back. To avoid their symptoms most people identified as having Pattern One pain would rather walk than stand and would rather stand than sit.

Pattern Three is far less common than Patterns One or Two. It represents constant pain that is more intense in the arm or leg than it is near the spine. In other respects it is similar to Pattern One: aggravated by forward bending, developing gradually over several hours or days, and continuing for weeks or even months at a time. When carefully considering their own symptoms, only one out of every ten neck or back pain sufferers qualifies as Pattern Three.

Pattern Four in the neck describes pain that can occur along the spine as well as spread into the arm. Symptoms in the upper limbs must be associated with spasticity in the legs. Pattern Four in the cervical spine is the only mechanical pattern which does not respond readily to posture correction and exercise. Its management requires close medical supervision and is not discussed in this book.

In the lumbar spine, Pattern Four is typified by leg dominant symptoms aggravated by activity and relieved by rest and a change in position. Like Pattern Three it is uncommon. Symptoms usually appear after the age of 50 and are heaviness or aching discomfort rather than severe stabbing pain.

Patients often complain that they are unable to walk for more than a few minutes before their legs begin to ache and feel weak. Sitting down relieves the problem, allowing them to resume walking and repeat the cycle. Pain control, the principle in the other three patterns, is not an issue since the symptoms subside as soon as the activity ceases. For people with Pattern Four the challenge is to raise their functional limits.

Although there is still some disagreement, most experts accept that Patterns One and Two are caused by irritation within the discs or small joints themselves. Pattern Three, commonly called "sciatica" in the leg, is believed to result from a bulging disc pressing directly on a nerve root. Pattern Four is probably produced by bony projections around the walls of a small spinal canal, choking the nerves and cutting off their normal blood supply. Whatever the theory, the patterns of pain remain.

You may be reassured to learn that your problem is no more ominous than a worn joint. But knowledge alone cannot stop the pain. To do that you must recognize your own pattern of pain, and employ the correct postures and exercises for your type of trouble.

Before practising the methods described in this book you should be familiar with a phenomenon called "centralization"—a shift in the location of pain following pain-control exercises or assuming the proper position. The more effective your routine, the closer your pain recedes to the center of your neck or low back. Centralization was described over 30 years ago by Robin McKenzie, a physiotherapist from New Zealand.

"Referred pain" from the cervical spine spreads first across the back of the neck, downward from the base of the skull. Next, it travels across the top of the shoulders and into the upper arms. At about the same time the pain radiates further down the back along the inner borders of the shoulder blades. A headache can climb across the top of the skull and lodge in the forehead and behind the eyes. Centralization is the reversal of this spread. Pain retreats down from the skull, up from the shoulder blades and back along the top of the shoulders until it resides only along the back of the neck.

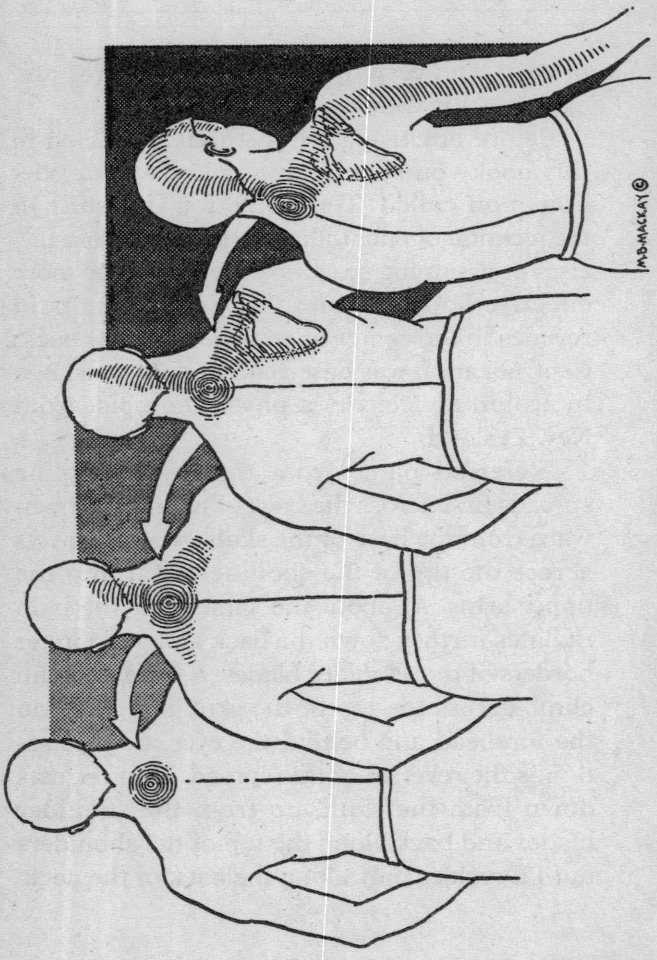
M.D.MACKAY ©

In the lumbar spine, mechanical pain refers first across the top of the pelvis then into the buttocks and down the back of the legs. It usually invades the thigh above the knee, but can advance as far as the foot. The pain can radiate around the trunk and cause aching in the groin and genitals. Centralization draws the pain from the front of the body and up from the legs and buttocks, shifting it to the center of the back below the waist.

Centralization is a positive sign. This may be hard to believe when you discover that centralization is often associated with an *increase* in pain. As the pain in the arm and leg decreases, the pain in the middle of your neck or back grows worse. Sometimes symptoms just vanish, but more often you will have to endure a brief period of discomfort before all your pain disappears.

Exercises, even as simple as those described here can produce a discomfort of their own. Separating the symptoms of your attack from

The progression to the right illustrates peripheralization. *Neck pain radiates to the shoulder, the shoulder blade, the head, and finally down the arm. The arrows to the left indicate* centralization, *a response to successful treatment that reverses the spread.*

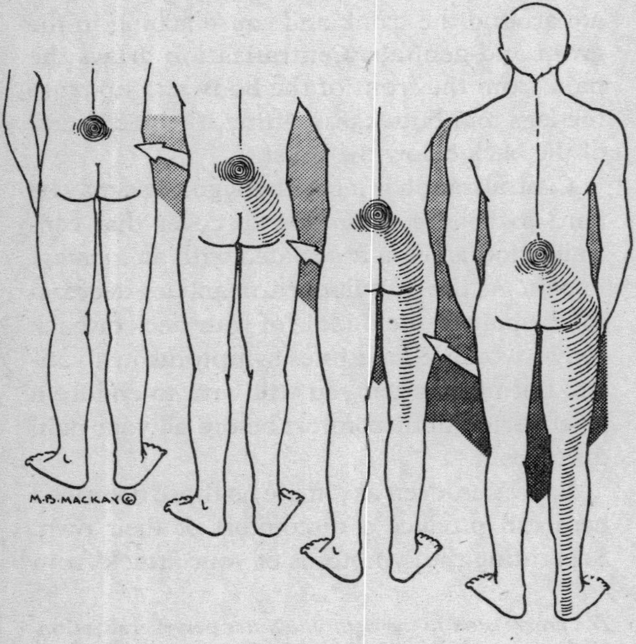
M.B.MACKAY©

the discomfort of exercise guides your program. The greater challenge may be discriminating the heightened pain of centralization from the accustomed pain of your acute episode.

Peripheralization, *the sequence moving to the right, advances the pain from the low back across the buttock and into the leg.* Centralization, *indicated by the arrows, returns pain to the spine where it may increase temporarily.*

Pattern Five

All pain is real. The amount of pain you feel results from many factors in addition to the mechanical problems in your neck or back.

For hundreds of years doctors believed that pains were created throughout the body, and the messages, like voices over a telephone, were sent to the brain. We understand now that although the signals of trouble can originate anywhere, they do not become pain until processed in the spinal cord or within the brain itself. A message of mechanical disturbance is the raw material; pain is the finished product. Converting the primary input into the perception of pain is a complex process and one that we have only recently begun to unravel. We know that the severity of the pain can be influenced greatly by fear, fatigue or preconceived expectations; by factors having nothing to do with the original physical injury. The process of pain production can be defective, creating intense agony in response to a trivial message.

For patients with Pattern Five the actual problem is the pain itself, not the extent of the physical damage. The characteristics of Pattern Five pain are quite different from those of the other four groups. Pattern Five tends to be a chronic condition, and although it occasionally begins shortly after the onset of symptoms, typically it is not apparent for several weeks or months. The clear reproducible picture of a mechanical pattern is absent. The elements of this pattern vary widely and often change over time. Symptoms migrate and the array of complaints expands to involve areas having no direct physical connection to the original problem.

Sleep appears to be controlled by the same neural functions or the same areas of the brain that create pain, so people with Pattern Five do not sleep well. They spend many long, uncomfortable hours during the night lying awake only to doze off during the day. Disruption of the normal sleep pattern produces a fatigue that accentuates the pain, further impairs the ability to rest, and creates a downward spiral.

The chronic pain of Pattern Five may impair sexual function, disrupt relationships, and produce an overwhelming sense of isolation and helplessness. It can induce depression, anxiety or hostility, emotions that further magnify the pain.

Individuals suffering Pattern Five symptoms often strenuously resist any implication that the problem is one of pain perception. They become obsessed with discovering the "real" cause of the pain, and when their doctor fails to identify a specific anatomical source they move on, always in search of a physical answer. Multiple medical opinions are inevitably accompanied by redundant investigations. Rather than establishing the lack of a physical problem, repeated failure to identify a mechanical source only convinces the sufferer of the complexity of the situation, and the inadequacy of the medical approach. This belief is strengthened by the inability of pain-killing medication and routine treatment to reduce the misery.

Pattern Five is perpetuated by the development of pain-centered behaviour. Pain becomes the determining factor in the sufferer's life, the basis for every choice or decision. This eccentric conduct demands justification, and there is no better validation than the regular use of pain medication. But since the sources of Pattern Five pain, improper processing and abnormal perception, lie beyond the reach of the medication, the pills don't work. The frequent response, both by the patient and the physician, is to increase the dose or add another drug. Reversing this destructive course is one of the principle goals in the management of Pattern Five.

Since we cannot directly attack the source of the pain, treatment is necessarily secondhand and often prolonged. Pain is a totally personal experience, difficult to analyze and impossible to isolate. Your feeling of pain is inseparable from your innate response. It is the magnitude of this response, your suffering and disability, that determines your behaviour, and it is your behaviour, the only visible manifestation of your pain, that gives any access to treatment.

Conquering Pattern Five is more difficult than overcoming one of the four mechanical patterns. Because the perception of pain has itself become the paramount problem, shifting the focus must be the principal treatment. This shift can not be accomplished simply by attempting to disregard the pain. In order to ignore it you must first acknowledge it, and that very acknowledgment reinforces your awareness. "Learn to live with your pain" is poor advice.

Something must replace the primacy of pain. There must be substitution. In a personal struggle against Pattern Five, the best replacement is activity—activity without relation to pain. Pain dictates behaviour. It is possible to reverse the process, to enable behaviour to dictate and ultimately annihilate pain. The first and most difficult step is to disconnect behaviour from pain. Remove pain as the decision maker and there is room to introduce alternatives, targets based on time, distance or a number of repetitions. These functional goals must be achievable. The initial mark is set well below the pain-imposed limit, then cautiously but invariably advanced without regard to the discomfort. Accomplishment must be measured. The record of progress is an essential weapon for success. The documented level of activity becomes incompatible with the existing level of pain. The dilemma forces a choice; either the activity is not possible because of the pain or the pain cannot exist with the history of function. The latter conclusion will result in a seemingly miraculous recovery.

Don't be fooled. A sudden disappearance of pain may follow weeks of diligent effort, weeks during which every activity hurts.

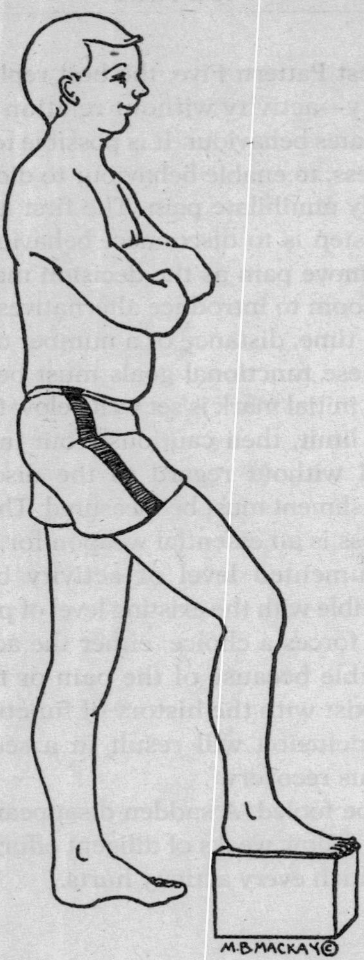
M.B.MACKAY©

YOUR PROGRAM FOR NECK PAIN RELIEF

Posture

It is difficult to change the position of your neck without changing the posture of your entire back. Standing and sitting with your lower spine slumped forward guarantees that you will bend your neck forward as well. It is no help to balance your head above your shoulders while your shoulders droop towards your knees. Correcting posture in the neck begins with correcting posture along the length of your spine.

While Standing

Most of us stand with our shoulders rounded and our chins thrust forward. Prolonged standing leads us to slouch, increasing the curve in the low back, sagging the shoulders and

The curve of the neck and low back is balanced by standing with one foot on a step. Periodically changing feet extends the duration of postural pain control.

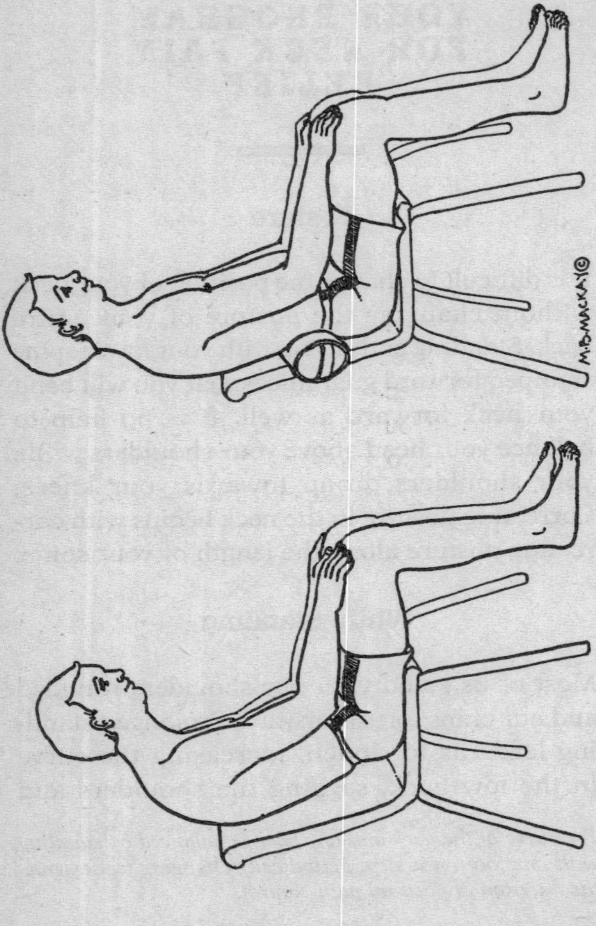
M.B.MACKAY©

pushing the head out. To change this posture you must first create the proper degree of arch in the low back, technically called "lordosis".

Placing one foot up on a step or stool puts the low back into a position of relaxed lordosis. This is the secret of the brass rail in the stand-up bar. Altering the position of the lumbar spine automatically changes the position of the shoulders, which then changes the posture of the head creating the desired forward curvature of the neck, cervical lordosis.

A similar effect can be achieved by "standing tall". Tighten your buttocks, suck in your stomach and raise your chest. This semblance of a military posture squares your shoulders and lifts your head but it requires sustained physical exertion.

While Sitting

The tendency to slouch or slump is even greater when you sit. Sink into a soft chair or bend forward over a desk and the lumbar spine

Sitting often creates a loss of lumbar lordosis associated with a head forward posture. By restoring the curve to the low back, a large lumber roll automatically improves the position of the cervical spine.

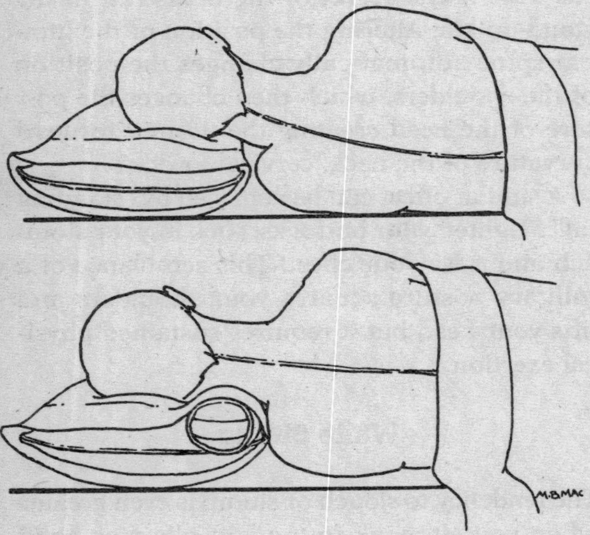
M.B.MAC

invariably loses its lordosis. Without a forward curve in the low back it is impossible to have proper cervical posture.

Providing the couch or chair will let you sit up straight, you can briefly recover your lumbar lordosis through conscious effort. For longer periods, the use of a lumbar support is essential. A lumbar roll, three to five inches (7½ to 12½ centimeters) in diameter, placed at waist level will push the lumbar spine into the desired position.

Begin by placing your buttocks against the back of your chair to gain the maximum effect. Once the lumbar spine is positioned properly, the shoulders, neck and head will follow and cervical lordosis will be restored.

While Lying

Lying down makes the position of the entire spine less important. In the recumbent position,

Lacking support, the neck sags between the head and shoulders. A neck roll or folded towel in the pillow case supports the cervical spine and provides postural pain relief. Many people fail at pain control because the cervical roll is too small. The roll must be large enough to provide full support and, at first, that can be uncomfortable.

postural strain occurs principally because the neck hangs unsupported between the head and shoulders like a clothesline between two poles. Elevating the sagging cervical spine requires external support and a rolled towel inside the pillow case may be all that is necessary. As you lie on your side the towel fills the gap between your ear and the point of your shoulder. The size of the roll depends upon the amount of space to be filled; the commonest mistake is to make the roll too small. The correct thickness should provide almost immediate pain relief.

Exercises for Neck Pain

Proper posture passively corrects the position of the head. Pain control exercise accomplishes the same thing through active movement.

Ordinarily, an exercise puts your spine through a greater range of movement and produces more rapid pain control, but even the most effective exercise cannot overcome the negative effects of prolonged poor posture.

Exercises should be performed as often as necessary to subdue your pain. Five to fifteen repetitions every hour or two is recommended. The precise routine will depend upon its effect.

Pain control exercises will often centralize your pain, moving it from your head, arm, shoulder blade or top of your shoulder to the middle of your neck. Although the central pain may increase temporarily, this is a positive result. You should reconsider the pain control exercises you have chosen only when your *typical* symptoms increase, or when your pain moves farther down your back or arm.

All pain control exercises should be performed in a slow, controlled fashion. Throwing your head forward or backward may gain you a few more degrees of movement but can increase your pain.

A rhythm can be established by slowly repeating to yourself "pressure on ... pressure off" with each movement.

It is easiest to learn most neck pain control exercises sitting down. To be sure that your spine is well supported, slide your buttocks against the back of the chair.

This is one time you don't need your lumbar roll. Too much support shifts the center of movement down into the lumbar spine and inhibits cervical motion. The back of the chair should extend no higher than your shoulder blades, allowing you to draw your shoulders back without obstruction. Padding the chair back with a towel or thin pillow may make it more comfortable.

Lying on your back to perform these exercises limits the accessible range of movement. This supine posture is useful when the neck pain is so acute that even a slight exaggeration of the correct maneuver intensifies the pain.

PATTERN ONE —NECK

While Standing

Most neck pain results from a head forward posture. The pain control maneuver requires an exercise called *retraction*. While looking forward, draw your head slowly backward so that your ears are directly above your shoulders. At first many people nod up or down instead of retracting. Imagine that your chin is sliding along the top of a table and practice until the movement follows a straight line. Done properly this exercise stretches the tight tissues at the base of your skull and increases motion in the lower part of your neck. You may experience a feeling of strain in one or both areas.

When you have drawn your head backward as far as it can go, relax and let it slide forward again. You may find it easier to perform a full retraction by lightly pressing the fingers of one hand on your chin. The pressure does not replace the action of the neck muscles, but it

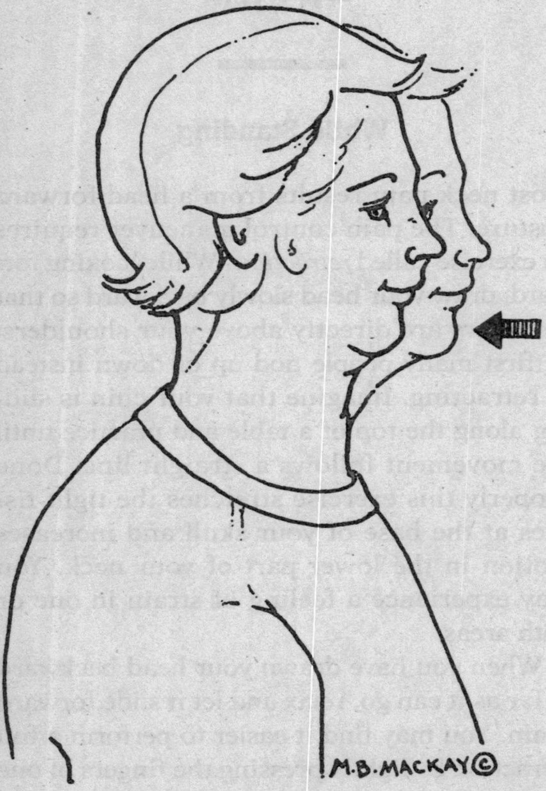
M.B. MACKAY©

seems to guide the movement, keeping it level and gaining a greater range.

Most people find it difficult to learn retraction while standing. It is easy to rock through the hips and lower back, and difficult to focus movement within the cervical spine. Practice standing retractions with your back against a wall to prevent additional movement. For many, the exercise is best learned while sitting.

While Sitting

By immobilizing the rest of your spine, retraction is isolated to the neck. The strain sensation is frequently stronger because movement is more pronounced.

Adding a backward roll of the shoulders increases the available range of movement. As you retract your head, press your fingertips lightly against your chin and keep your eyes level. If the exercise is performed correctly you will feel your chest rise.

Beyond retraction is extension—bending the neck backward to look up. If retraction helps,

Retraction *means drawing the head backward while keeping the eyes level. Guiding the chin with the finger tips helps avoid an unwanted up and down movement.*

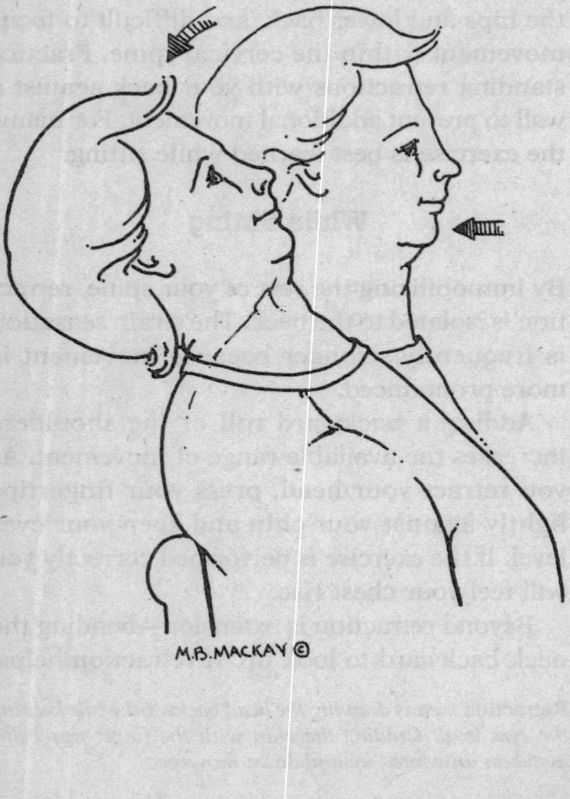
M.B.MACKAY ©

you may wish to proceed to this next step. Holding the retracted position, raise your chin and tilt your head. Don't let your chin come forward.

As you arch backwards, turn your head slightly from side to side. When you have gone as far as you can, relax in that position for a moment, straighten up and start again.

While Lying

As you lie without a pillow, your head is resting at the same level of your shoulders but your neck still has its lordosis, its forward curve. Stare at a point on the ceiling, press your head backward against the mattress, and draw your chin down. You should be able to decrease the cervical curve without nodding. Hold the position for a moment or two and then release, allowing your chin to come forward and your neck to arch. You can check that you are performing this exercise correctly by placing one hand behind your neck to feel the changes in pressure.

Adding extension *after full* retraction *may decrease Pattern One neck pain. Attempt extension when retraction alone affords merely partial relief.*

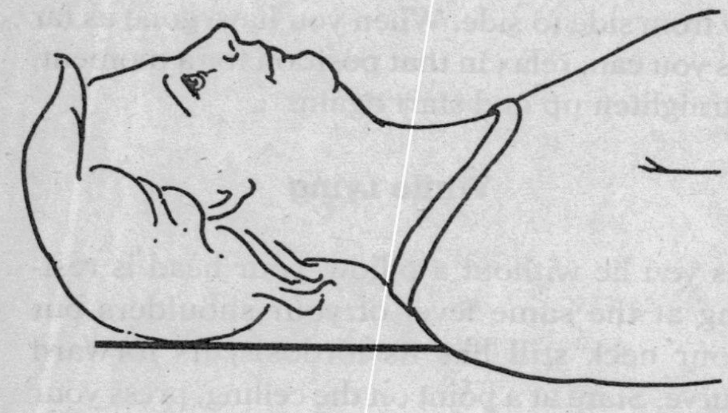
M.B.MACKAY©

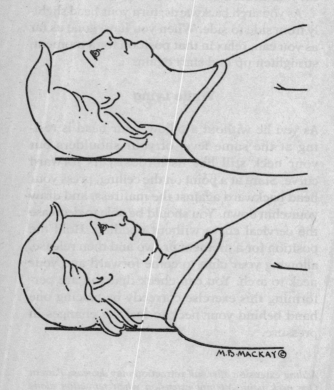

As with all pain control exercises, a positive response is a shift of the pain toward the middle of the neck, or better still, immediate abolition of the symptoms. An increase in the typical pain or symptoms moving away from the mid-line is an indication to stop.

Because the supine position is used only in the most acute circumstances, even minute modifications of position or range can have profound effects. Don't be afraid to experiment; even in this extreme situation you cannot cause harm.

If retraction is beneficial but some pain remains, try extension. Lie on your back at the end of the bed so that your head and shoulders stick out over the edge. Before you move into this position place one hand behind your head for support. Begin with retraction then gradually lower your head. When you have gone as far as you can, tip your head backward. Keep turning your head a little to each side as you extend. If your pain diminishes hang there for several seconds then use your hand to raise yourself back to the neutral position.

Enough cervical lordosis remains while lying to allow retraction. *The reduction in the available range of movement makes this combination particularly useful for acute neck pain or headache control.*

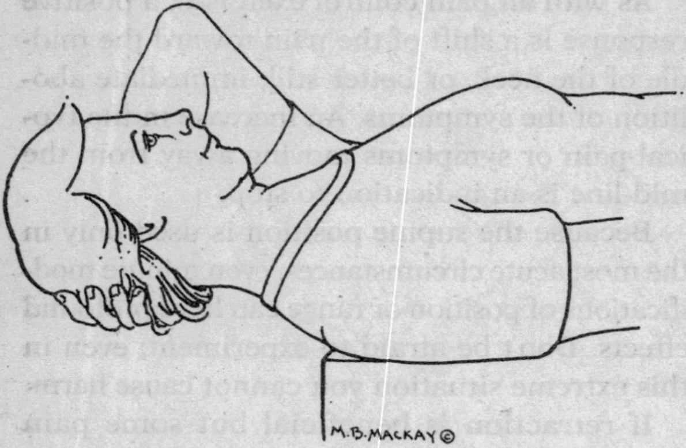
M.B.MACKAY ©

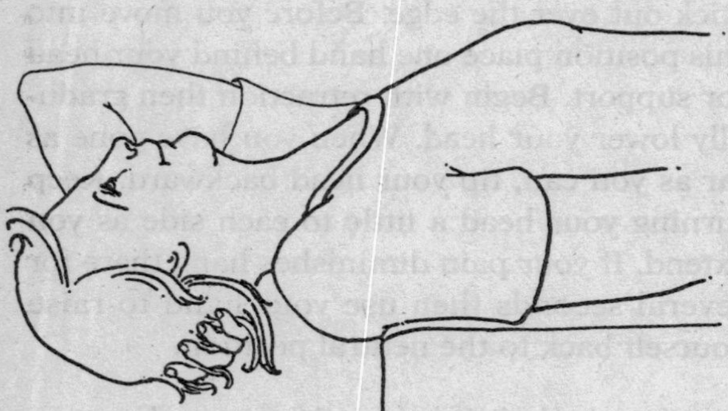
M.B.MACKAY ©

Pattern One responds to retraction and extension and is increased by forward bending, so try to lie flat between the exercise repetitions. If possible, don't use a pillow. For some people, however, the head forward posture is so fixed that a small pillow or folded towel is required to avoid increasing the pain.

Retraction *while lying is increased when the head and neck project beyond the end of the bed. Support the head and slowly draw the chin down.* (top)

Gravity adds an element of traction to retraction and extension while lying. If the position feels secure and comfortable, remove the hand for a few moments but use it again to raise the head. (bottom)

M.B.MACKAY©

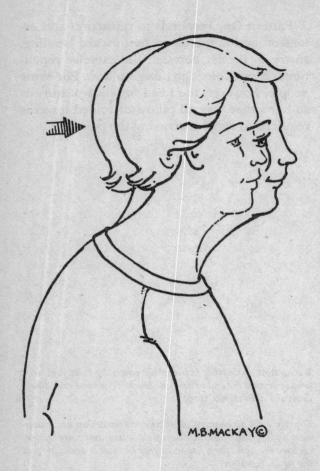

PATTERN TWO —NECK

While Standing

Because this pattern of neck pain is often sudden in onset and short in duration, relieving the episode is seldom difficult. The pain is usually associated with a specific extension movement, looking up at the ceiling for example, and pain control may be as simple a dropping your chin onto your chest. Few repetitions, often no more than four or five, should be required for relief.

A similar but slightly more complex flexion movement is *protraction*. This movement is the reverse of the maneuver for Pattern One. Gently push your head forward, keeping your eyes level and your chin parallel to the floor. Push to the point of strain then allow your head to shift back over your shoulders. Only a few repetitions should be required to reduce the pain.

Protraction *thrusts the chin forward but keeps the head level. Look straight ahead and feel the pressure in the back of the neck at the base of the skull.*

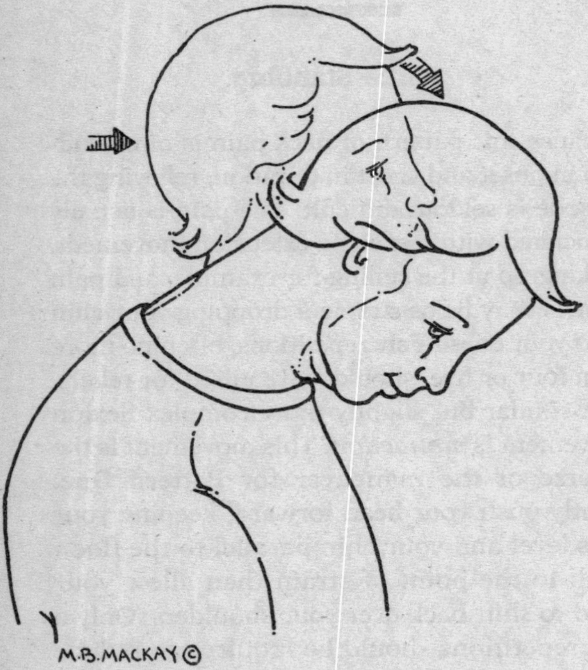
M.B.MACKAY ©

As with most neck pain control exercises, protraction is best learned while sitting, and then may be adapted to the standing position.

While Sitting

Flexion and protraction are accomplished easily in the sitting position. Flexion can be increased by interlocking your fingers, keeping your elbows pointing forward, and then placing your hands behind your head. As your chin drops to your chest, the weight of your arms and, perhaps, a gentle downward pull, increases the effect. Pain relief should require few repetitions.

While Lying

Pain control for Pattern Two seldom requires exercise in the recumbent position. Resting your head on a soft pillow to flex your neck and then gently raising your chin toward your chest may be helpful.

Combining flexion *with* protraction *may reduce Pattern Two neck symptoms. Additional pressure can be applied by clasping the hands behind the head. Progress only when protraction alone provides imcomplete pain control.*

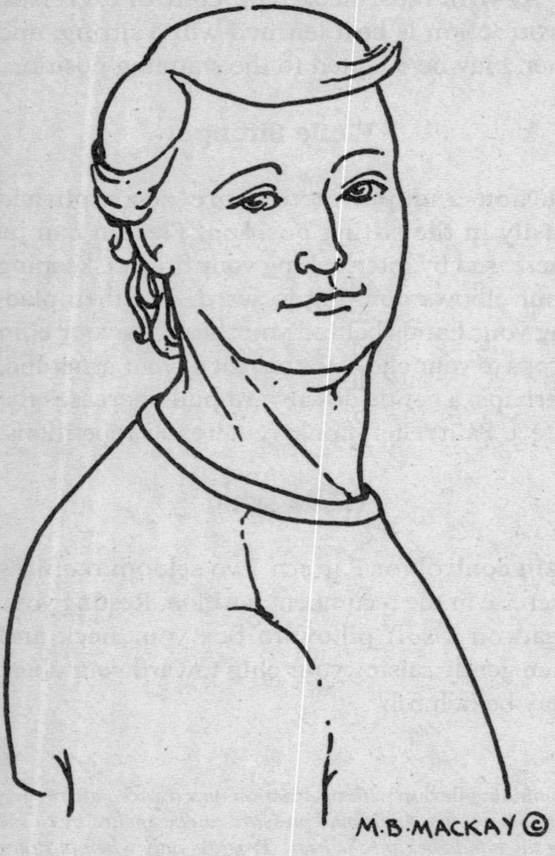
M·B·MACKAY ©

PATTERN THREE —NECK

While Standing

Most people who suffer Pattern Three neck pain where the dominant pain is actually in the arm and not in the neck, respond to the retraction exercise described for Pattern One. Generally, the response is slower and the centralization effect is more pronounced. Sustained retraction seems more effective than repetitive movement. To successfully control Pattern Three, retraction is often combined with an additional movement such as side bending or rotation.

Since each situation is different, experiment with a number of combinations until you find the one that most rapidly reduces your pain. There is no danger; you cannot injure your spine with these simple pain control maneuvers.

In a few cases pain control requires a combination of movements. Turning the head slightly to one side may enhance pain reduction. Retraction *increases the range of* rotation.

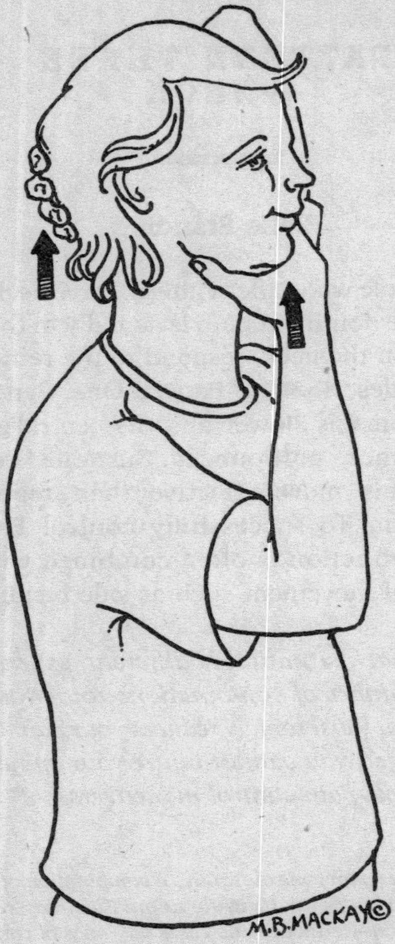
M.B.MACKAY©

While Sitting

The pain control exercises in sitting for Pattern Three are similar to those for Pattern One. Holding a position rather than using repetitive movement is usually more effective.

Sometimes Pattern Three responds to brief periods of self-traction, but unfortunately, the relief usually lasts only as long as the traction is maintained. Place the palm of one hand under your chin and push up. Grip the back of your head with the other hand and pull up. A slight stretch of the neck can produce a considerable reduction in typical arm pain. Retracting or rotating your head as you apply traction may magnify the beneficial effects.

While Lying

There is no difference in the exercises for Pattern Three and those for Pattern One. As always, Pattern Three responds more consistently to sustained posture than to repetitive movement.

Manual traction may offer short-term relief. Experiment by adding retraction, protraction, flexion, extension *or* rotation. *Unfortunately, the benefit usually lasts only as long as pressure is applied.*

Generally, symptoms lessen with retraction or extension, but forcing your neck into an extreme position can aggravate the arm pain. You may want to experiment with your head on a folded towel or thin pillow to locate the ideal resting posture. A roll under your neck prevents the cervical spine from sagging and can further diminish discomfort.

HEADACHE

Because headaches can be so debilitating they deserve a section of their own. Some people suffer headaches as part of their original neck pain. Others experience them for the first time while attempting a control maneuver for pain in another location, a maneuver that stretches tight tissues in the neck and sets off this unwanted reaction.

Controlling mechanical headaches is a strategy of small movements. An extra centimeter of protraction or retraction may make the difference .

The key is finding the "escape position", a posture that can almost magically abolish the headache. Start by slowly moving your head forward into protraction. Stop at the point you feel the headache increase. You may not have to move very far. Now move backward into retraction. Stop when the pain intensifies. You have now identified the margins of your escape position. Move cautiously. The range may be small and it's possible to slide right through the position and never know it.

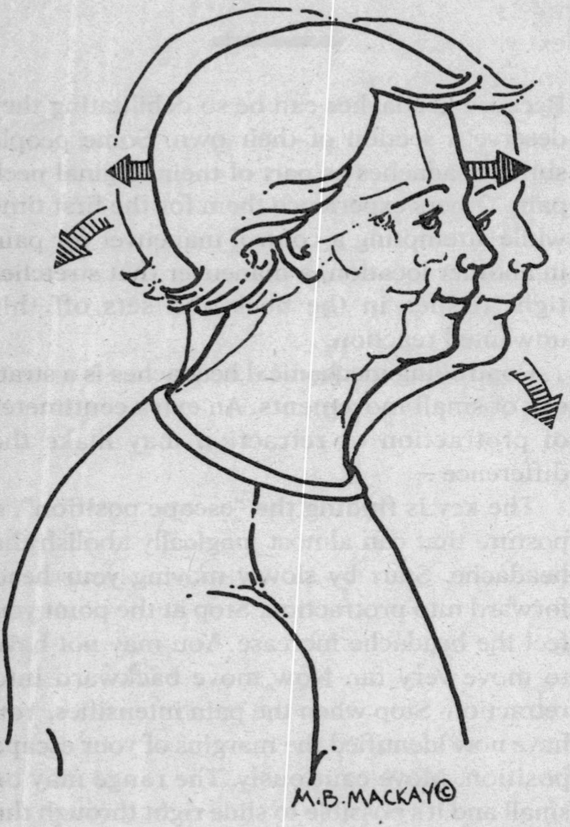
M.B.MACKAY©

Once you can identify a posture that centralizes or even extinguishes the headache, the next step is to expand that pain-free zone by gently pushing out the boundaries. Glide your head forward until the pain returns. Hold a position just beyond the pain-free limit and nod gently. Nodding stretches the tight tissues and increases the range. If you can influence your typical pain you are working on the correct area. Your pain will determine the amount of stretching you can accomplish at a single try. Move in the opposite direction and nod to enlarge the area backward. Stay with small movements; stretching too fast causes too much pain.

While Standing

Few people can control mechanical headaches while standing because of the weight of the head in the upright position and the necessary precision of the exercises.

Enlarge the headache-escape position by combining protraction *and* retraction *with* nods. *Move forward just beyond the limits of the pain-free zone, then slowly nod to increase the available range. Repeat the same maneuver moving backwards.*

While Sitting

Careful attention to the lumbar support may produce enough change in the cervical posture to reduce the headache. Use a lumbar roll and vary its thickness or adjust your distance from the back of the chair for maximum benefit. Adding a backward shift of the shoulders is seldom necessary.

While Lying

Headache control is most potent lying down. Locate and maintain the escape position with a small pillow or by supporting the head with folded towels. The proper thickness is critical; move up or down one fold at a time. Establish and slowly expand the pain-free region with protraction, retraction and nods.

WHIPLASH

Many people are surprised to learn that "whiplash" is not a medical diagnosis. The term refers only to the manner of injury, not to the injury itself.

Although whiplash can be caused in a variety of ways, the best-known example is a rear end automobile collision. Whiplash describes the neck movement as the head is thrown back and forth. Even a velocity as low as six to eight kilometers per hour has an effect greater than four times the force of gravity. At impact the occupant in a car seat is driven forward at the same rate as the vehicle. Because nothing pushes the head, it remains behind in its original position. This tendency for something to remain at rest until affected by an external force is called "inertia". It's the same reason a ball in the middle of the floor does not begin rolling by itself. When the body moves forward it pulls the head along. While the head lags behind the shoulders, the neck arches backward forcing the cervical spine beyond its normal range, stretching muscles and ligaments, and putting pressure on the interlock-

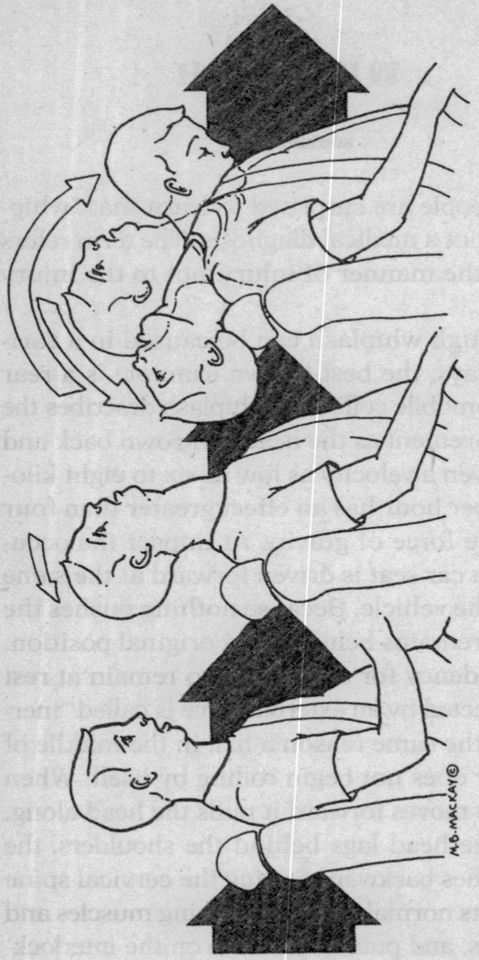
M.B. MACKAY©

ing joints. Then, the elastic nature of the spine pulls the head forward, sometimes with enough force to bounce the chin off the chest. The whole cycle can be repeated two or three times.

Recent studies have shown that the same event, a rear end collision, may produce a different mechanism of injury. Impact can lift the occupant out of the seat. The head flies up, stretching the neck. Instead of whipping back and forth, the force acts up and down pulling on the neck then slamming the weight of the head down against the cushioning discs.

With two different mechanisms damaging structures in the neck, it is hardly surprising that the causes of pain vary considerably. Muscles may tear. Ligaments may rupture. Portions of the disc wall may give way or you can sprain a joint between the vertebrae. Fortunately, the injury is usually minimal, a small bruise in the muscle, for example. A few cases of whiplash can involve fractures, dislocations or trauma to the nervous system.

The dark arrow represents the sudden advance of the vehicle. As the body is pushed forward, the head remains behind and arches back over the seat. An improperly placed head support can actually increase the effect. Recoil snaps the head forward with enough force to bounce the chin off the chest.

Complicating this wide range of possible problems is the fact that they usually occur in combination, with no one location being the only source of pain. No wonder the concept of whiplash creates such controversy. From a diagnostic perspective the word can mean almost anything.

Receiving a whiplash can be a frightening experience. Pain at a time of high stress is increased by resentment and confrontation. Initially, it may be impossible to believe that most people can expect a rapid recovery and will return to normal function in a short time. Statistics clearly show, however, that the majority will be better within a few weeks and that over 98 percent will recover fully within one year. The rate of improvement varies, of course, with the severity of the original injury and your body's natural rate of healing.

In spite of its diversity, every pattern of pain produced by the mechanism of whiplash can be grouped into one of the patterns described in this book. Even here treatment is directed at eliminating symptoms without immediate regard for the specific physical site of the pain. Pain control in the acute phase relies on maneuvers appropriate to the dominant pattern. Experimentation is acceptable and worthwhile. Except for fractures, dislocated joints or injuries to the spinal nerves, all of which are readily identifiable on a post-injury medical assessment, any physical damage caused by the accident will not increase with early resumption of normal movement. More than any other back or neck pain sufferer, the whiplash victim must be aware that hurt does not necessarily indicate harm.

Although neck pain, compounded by the aggravation of a motor vehicle accident, is an emotionally charged experience, its physical aspects are similar to the more mundane sprained ankle. The soft tissues, muscles and ligaments bear the brunt of the trauma but usually preserve joint stability. Healing proceeds rapidly in these tissues, restoring 90 percent of their intact strength within six weeks. The quality of healing improves significantly if the involved structures are moved gently within the normal range during the early stages of recovery. In both the neck and the ankle, the frequent long-term problem is stiffness more than stability. Following injury the body's first response is an outpouring of fluid through the walls of local blood vessels into the damaged tissue. The medical term for this fluid is "edema". While edema formation is natural and enhances the rapid delivery of healing elements, its persistence is counter-productive. "Edema is glue". Imagine you spill a soft drink on the pages of this book. Clean it off without delay and the book may suffer no lasting damage. Let it dry and the pages can stick together permanently. The tissue planes in your neck are similar to the pages of the book. They are designed to slide across each other to allow free movement. Stick them together and the movement is lost. Once the glue has set, try to pull the tissues apart and it hurts. Restoring lost movement can be a formidable task. Moving the tissues through their normal range within hours of the accident squeezes the edema out, allowing it to provide benefit without causing lasting problems.

Perhaps the most insidious promoter of long-term loss of movement in the neck is the soft cervical collar. The collar prevents movement, allows persistent edema formation and promotes an attitude of helplessness. Active movement during the first two or three days after a whiplash injury to reduce the build up of tissue fluid is now recognized as a critical step in establishing rapid recovery. The soft collar cannot stabilize the neck and so is of no value in the rare cases of fracture or joint disruption, and it retards recovery in the overwhelming majority of cases suffering only degrees of soft tissue injury. For those with Pattern One pain the collar actually puts the neck in a position that increases the symptoms.

PAIN CONTROL AFTER WHIPLASH

Posture

Finding a position that reduces the strain on sore tissues is the first step in pain control. The neck is the upper portion of the spine and cannot be positioned properly without adjusting the posture in the rest of the back. Sitting with a lumbar roll, even if there is no back pain, can reduce symptoms in the neck.

Pattern One

Balancing the head above the shoulders with gentle retraction is often effective. Sitting with a support high against the back of the head provides protection and maintains correct posture. Lying down with a cervical roll along the lower edge of the pillow to keep the spine from sagging can provide the most relief of all.

Pattern Two

Letting your chin drop toward your chest or supporting your chin in your hands can decrease the pain. Once again, lying with the cervical roll works by preventing sag. Although the direction of pain production is different, the benefit of keeping the spine balanced is the same.

Pattern Three

Constant arm-dominant pain after a whiplash injury is unusual and may represent substantial damage to the disc. Pain control through retraction, a head rest and a cervical roll can be helpful but a professional evaluation of the situation is advisable.

PAIN CONTROL AFTER WHIPLASH

Exercise

Because of the recent soft tissue injury, pain control movements should be gentle and limited in extent. Starting aggressively will cause no harm but neither will it control the symptoms. Small, frequent neck movements within the normal range retard the formation of excessive edema, improve the strength and flexibility of the healing tissues and reduce the short-term pain. Start slowly. A decrease in your symptoms is the best indicator of an exercise's effectiveness.

PATTERN ONE —WHIPLASH

While Standing

It is difficult to learn retraction in standing even when you are pain free. The pain and muscle spasm following whiplash generally render pain control when standing ineffective.

While Sitting

Be sure that your spine is well supported against the back of a chair. Many people find that the use of a head rest adds a feeling of stability and makes the retraction exercise more comfortable. Naturally, the head rest also reduces the range of movement but, in the presence of newly injured tissue, this can aid pain control. Details of the retraction exercise are covered on page 37.

While Lying

Because the recumbent position eliminates the weight of the head pressing down on the neck, just lying down may reduce the pain. Retraction in lying reduces the available range and a soft pillow and cervical roll add a sense of stability. After a whiplash injury many people find it best to begin their exercise program lying on their backs. Details of retraction while lying are covered on page 39.

PATTERN TWO —WHIPLASH

While Standing

Gently flexing the head a few times may bring temporary relief, but if the whiplash has produced dizziness or lightheadedness the standing position is not the way to start.

While Sitting

Lowering the chin toward the chest can bring relief. Adding more pressure by clasping the hands behind the head is rarely helpful. Details of pain control with flexion while sitting are covered on page 47.

While Lying

The flexion exercise begins with the head on a soft but fairly thick pillow. Experiment by altering the starting position to increase or reduce the available range of movement. A small correction can dramatically heighten the exercise's effectiveness.

Because of the frequent combination of Pattern One and Pattern Two pain following the whiplash mechanism, many people do best with a combination of routines. Alternate between flexion and retraction but keep the amplitude of the movements low. If they are effective, repeat the exercises as frequently as possible, even several times an hour, employing five to ten repetitions per session.

PATTERN THREE —WHIPLASH

Pain control exercise for constant arm-dominant pain may be of little value. Techniques for dealing with Pattern Three are described on pages 49-51, but when these symptoms appear after a whiplash injury, professional assessment is recommended. Before jumping to the worst conclusion, however, carefully note the site of dominant pain. Both Patterns One and Two often radiate into the arm. It is only when pain below the shoulder is constant and unequivocally more intense than the discomfort along the spine that Pattern Three is a real possibility.

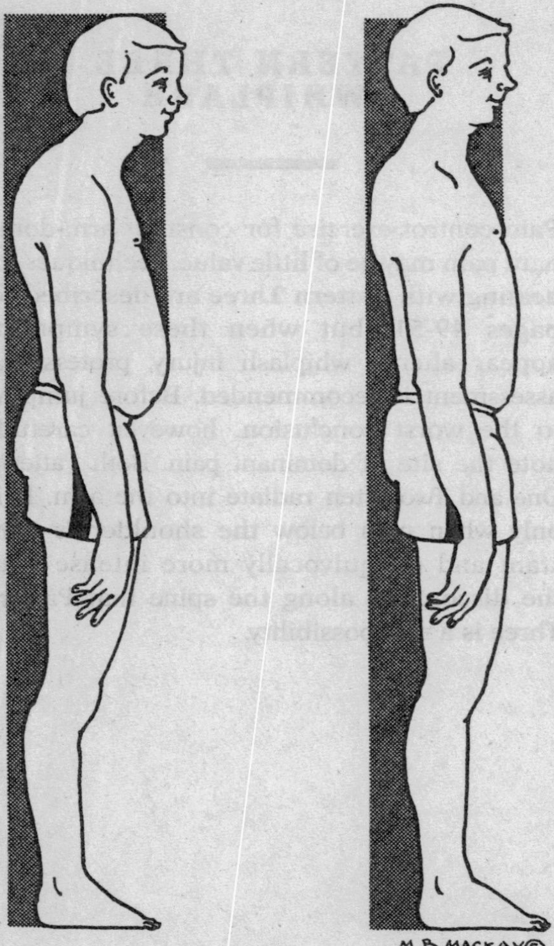
M.B.MACKAY©

YOUR PROGRAM FOR BACK PAIN RELIEF

Posture

Depending upon the pain pattern, the goal of proper posture is to increase or decrease the natural curve of the low back. The correct position will centralize, reduce or eliminate the typical pain. Paradoxically this posture may not feel comfortable. It's natural to confuse comfort with pain control. Comfort can be defined as "a state of ease" but the positions required for pain control may be too extreme to be pleasant. Shortly before they realize that the typical pain has disappeared, many people remark that their new posture feels wrong. This isn't surprising when you understand that most back pain results from a habit of bad posture and that breaking any habit is difficult.

Squaring the shoulders, drawing in the stomach and tensing the buttocks reduces an unwanted head forward position. Most people improve their neck posture involuntarily as they stand up.

While Standing

Most people arch their backs too much when they stand. The longer they stand while the shoulders droop and the abdomen bulges, the more pronounced the curve becomes. Improve your standing posture by drawing back your head, raising your chest, tightening your stomach and tensing your buttocks. Square your shoulders and for a moment or two balance lightly on the balls of your feet.

The same type of posture correction can be achieved with much less effort by standing with one foot up on a box, step or rail. Either foot will do. Change your posture frequently by alternating the position of your feet.

While Sitting

The common problem while sitting is too little lumbar lordosis. The solution is to increase rather than diminish the curve. Although you can improve your posture for short periods voluntarily, it is impossible for your muscles alone to hold the desired lumbar curve.

Correcting sitting posture requires the use of a lumbar support. Most stuffed furniture is woefully inadequate. Sagging into soft cushions guarantees trouble. Adding a lumbar roll that is swallowed by the upholstery offers no solution.

Begin with a firm, straight-backed chair—padded perhaps, but not over-stuffed. The back of the seat should recline about ten degrees and the seat itself should be wide enough for you to shift your weight easily. Your feet should reach the floor without a struggle and there should be no pressure on the back of your thighs. Arm rests are helpful for rising and for a momentary transfer of body weight from your buttocks to your shoulders.

To this "suitable" chair add extra low back support. Many people try a rolled towel, but that has several drawbacks. The towel seldom holds its shape and even when it does, it lacks portability. Just try to appear nonchalant with a beach towel over your arm on the subway in December. Commercially available lumbar rolls are more suitable but choosing the best design is not always obvious. It's not necessarily the one that feels best: it's the one that stops the pain. A three-to five-inch (7½ to 12½ centimeter) diameter foam core is usually effective. Many ready-made supports are too thin to produce the required amount of lumbar lordosis.

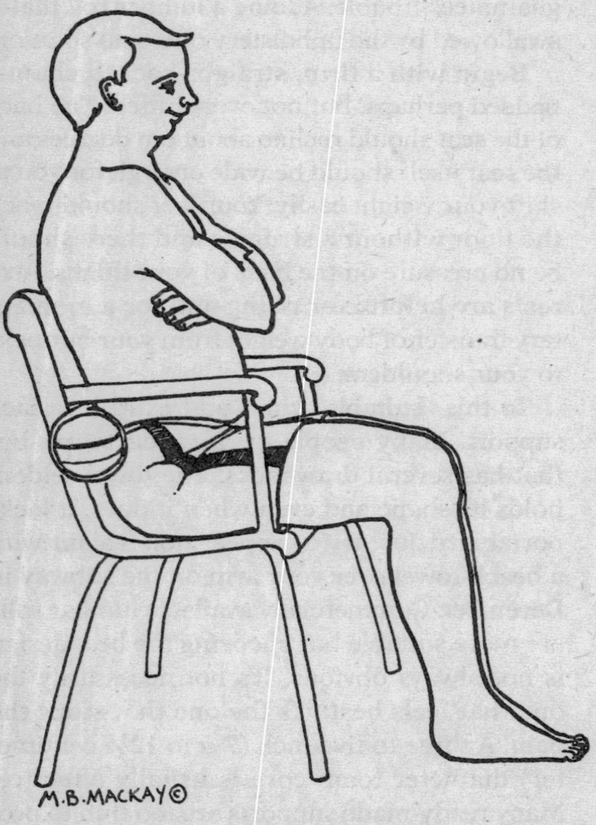
M.B.MACKAY©

People often prefer a model that feels natural over one that produces an effect. Their goal should be to change a typical posture into a corrective one. It's an issue of comfort versus pain control.

To use the support properly, slide your buttocks to the back of the seat. Place the roll at about belt level and arch backwards. If this position is too extreme, "cheat" by sliding your buttocks slightly forward. As the flexibility of your lumbar spine increases you will be able to move back.

Stand and move about as often as possible; pull over and get out of the car, get up from the desk and walk to the fax machine. No matter how effectively you modify the seat, prolonged sitting can still be a source of pain. Even sitting perfectly, thirty minutes is about the longest period you can expect to remain pain free without moving.

Many chairs lack adequate lumbar support. The addition of a lumbar roll reduces Pattern One low back pain. A chair with arms allows a brief transfer of weight to the shoulders giving the back a rest.

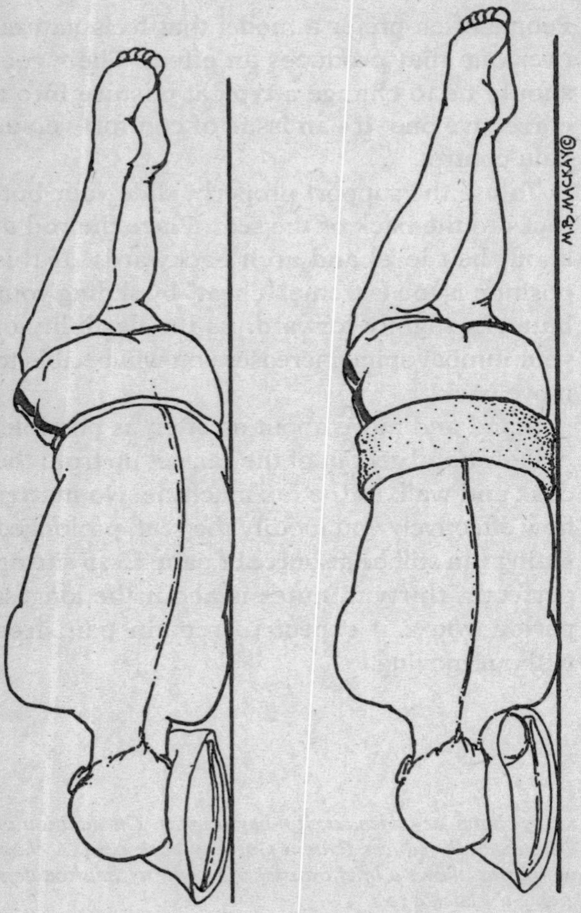
M.B. MACKAY©

While Lying

Removing upper body weight makes it easier to maintain the normal lumbar curve. Now the problem is the spine's tendency to sag as it travels unsupported between your chest and your pelvis. No matter the surface, filling the gap under your waist can be easily accomplished with a rolled towel.

To ensure that the support remains in the correct position it's better to wear the towel than to roll it up beneath you. Wrap the towel around the sash from a bathrobe or housecoat, leaving the ends of the sash free. Use them to tie the towel around your waist.

The size you require is the height necessary to lift your spine into a straight line when you lie on your side or to maintain the correct amount of lordosis when you lie on your back. Because a large roll looks silly, most people wind the towel roll too small. One size definitely does not fit all. The correct thickness is the

Wrapping a rolled towel around the waist supports the spine between the rib cage to the pelvis. The roll must raise the spine to a straight line and lying on a roll thick enough to have an effect may produce local discomfort. Success is measured by the reduction in typical pain.

one that reduces, eliminates, or at least centralizes the typical pain.

Wrapping your arms and legs around a large pillow is another aid to pain relief. Turning over twists the back, an unpleasant movement for a painful spine. Embracing the thick pillow allows you to move as a single unit without rotating your shoulders above your hips.

Exercises For Back Pain

Most low back pain is Pattern One and the rest is almost all Pattern Two. Patterns Three and Four are uncommon. When a combination of patterns exists, choose the exercise that attacks the dominant problem and be prepared to create a mixed program when necessary. Typically, the movements for pain control are roughly opposite to those producing pain.

Sitting loads the spine more than standing erect does, and this limits the effectiveness of some pain control exercises. Lying down removes the effect of gravity and makes these exercises very useful.

Pain control exercises should be repeated frequently throughout the day. A good starting point is ten repetitions every two hours. Alter the time interval and the number of repetitions as your pain dictates. Perform the exercises deliberately. Rushing ten repetitions gains you less than five repetitions performed carefully. Regular breathing adds relaxation and sets an appropriate pace.

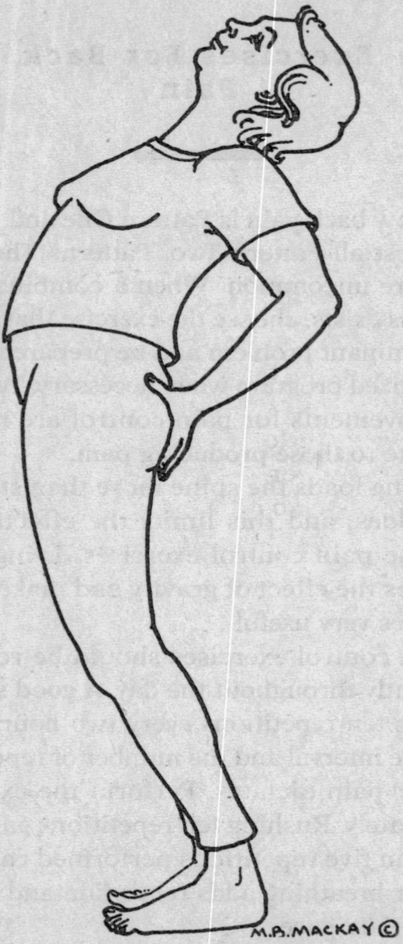
M.B. MACKAY ©

PATTERN ONE —BACK

While Standing

Standing up to arch backward is a natural reaction to prolonged sitting. As an exercise, the limitation is the amount of curve you can produce in your low back. Place your hands low on your buttocks and push your hips forward without bending your knees. Keep your head balanced above your shoulder; don't just arch your neck. Standing extensions can be repeated as often and with as many repetitions as necessary to control the typical pain.

While Sitting

To extend your lower spine actively from the sitting position requires a seat without a back. Take a firm grip with your hands to avoid toppling

Extension *while standing should focus on the lumbar spine. Keep the hips and knees locked. Avoid extending the neck. Placing the hands on the low back restricts the necessary movement, so push forward on the buttocks.*

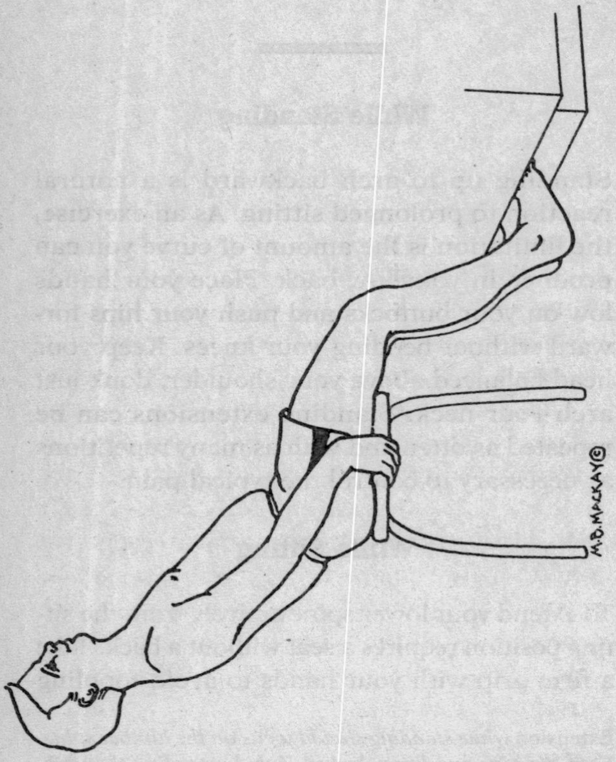
M.D.MACKAY©

over. Although extension in sitting has the advantage of eliminating unwanted movement in the hips and knees, most people find this an awkward exercise.

While Lying

The "sloppy push-up" is, for most people, the most effective exercise for Pattern One pain. Begin by lying on your stomach with your hands palms down, beside your shoulders. Push up, raising your trunk but keeping your hips down. Continue to push until your arms are straight and you can lock your elbows. Concentrate on letting your back sag. Hold briefly, "pressure on", and release, "pressure off".

Your performance and your range of movement will tend to improve with repetition. Start by pushing up only until the pain suggests you should stop. Relax and repeat. With each push-up you should be able to raise your shoulders higher until you can fully extend and lock your arms. As the arch in your back increases your pain should decrease.

Extension *while sitting fixes the pelvis and targets the low back but restricts the range of movement. Maintain balance by hooking the feet under a ledge.*

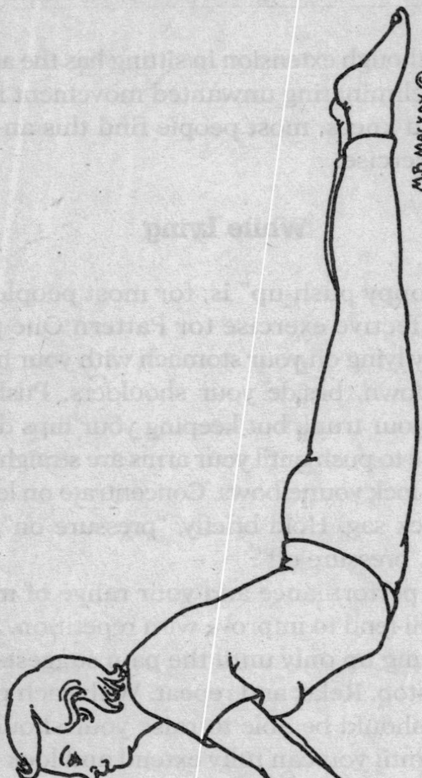
M.B. MACKAY ©

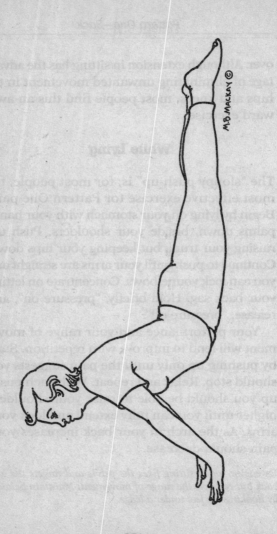

Some backs will not arch sufficiently to allow a complete push-up, and it is no help to raise your pelvis and lift your body from the knees up. This doesn't make your back move at all. Instead, start with your hands above your shoulders, beside your head. Now your arms can straighten fully with a reduced amount of back movement. As your ability improves, move your hands down.

Occasionally, the sloppy push-up will significantly reduce the pain but stop short of abolishing it altogether. In this case, further extension may produce a greater effect. Some people find it helpful to coordinate their breathing with the exercise. Breathe in before you start and breathe out at the top of the push-up. The added relaxation accentuates the sag in the low back. For a few people, holding the pelvis down increases the benefit. Try a belt or get help from your exercise partner.

Extension *while lying is the most effective exercise for Pattern One. It permits a full range of movement and works without gravity. Keep the hips down and concentrate on relaxing the low back. Adjust the height of the extension by altering the starting hand position; the closer to the shoulders, the greater the amount of extension.*

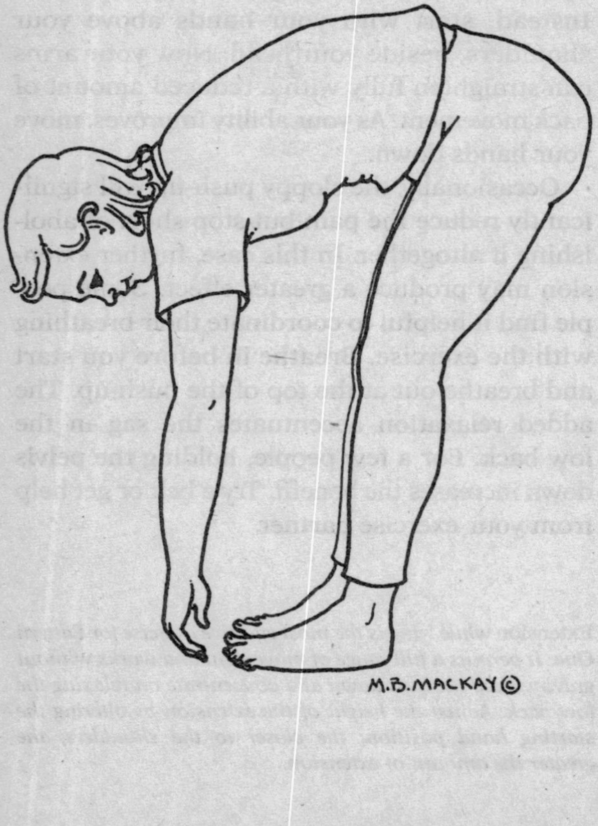
M.B. MACKAY ©

PATTERN TWO —BACK

While Standing

Ordinarily bending forward, flexion, reduces Pattern Two pain. Bend at the waist and let your hands drop towards your feet. Don't hurry and don't strain. The purpose is not to touch your toes but to relieve your pain.

Flexion *while standing is done slowly. The purpose is to stretch the spine, not touch the toes. Move under control; don't throw the upper body toward the floor.*

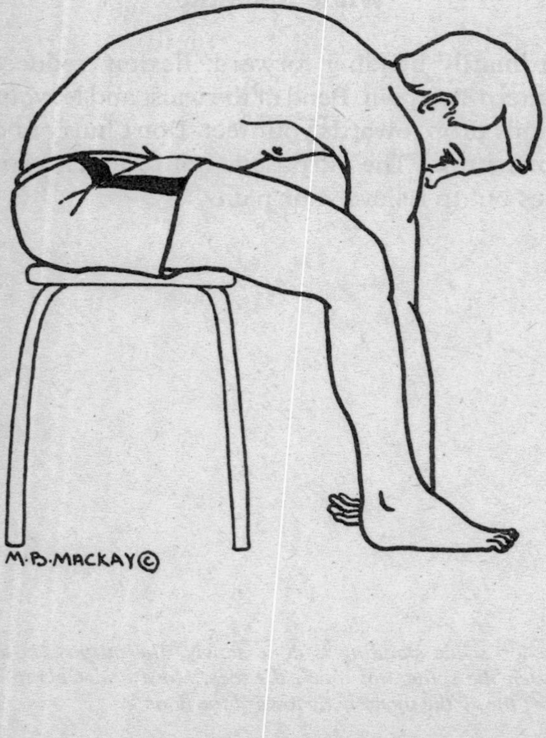
M.B.MACKAY©

While Sitting

Bend forward and let your chest slump toward your knees. Hold the position for a few moments then straighten up and do it again. If coming up hurts, put your hands on your knees and push yourself erect.

To make the exercise more difficult straighten your legs and slide your hands toward your ankles. This also stretches the hamstring muscles in the back of the thighs.

Flexion *while sitting allows a large range of movement, and fixing the pelvis forces flexion into the lower back. The degree of stretch is increased by extending the knees.*

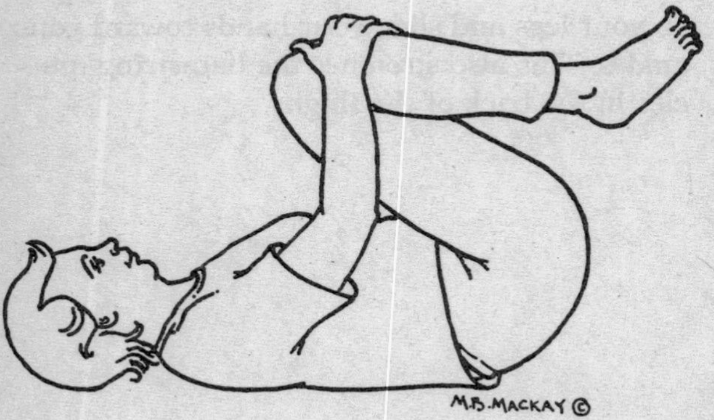
M.B.MACKAY ©

While Lying

Drawing both knees toward the chest flexes the lumbar spine. Exercising one leg at a time is much less effective since it isolates the hip and produces little back movement. Bend your knees and use your hands to pull your legs up. If your arms aren't long enough try pulling on the ends of a towel passed behind your thighs. Repeat five to ten times.

Drawing both knees toward the chest flexes the lumbar spine. Pulling up one knee at a time prevents rotation of the pelvis and stretches the hip rather than the back.

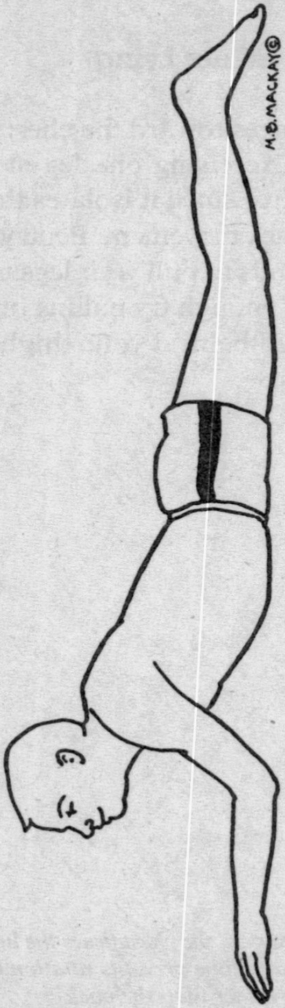
M.B.MACKAY©

PATTERN THREE

While Standing

People with Pattern Three, leg-dominant pain, rarely find relief while standing. Arching your back may help and it is a good idea to avoid bending forward, but the effective exercises are done lying down.

While Sitting

Most people with Pattern Three find it difficult to sit. Extension exercises are appropriate but rarely beneficial.

Prone lying on the elbows arches the low back. The amount of curve is determined by the position of the arms. For Patterns One and Three this position may produce centralization *as pain rises out of the leg and moves into the low back. In spite of a possible temporary increase in pain this is a sign of success.*

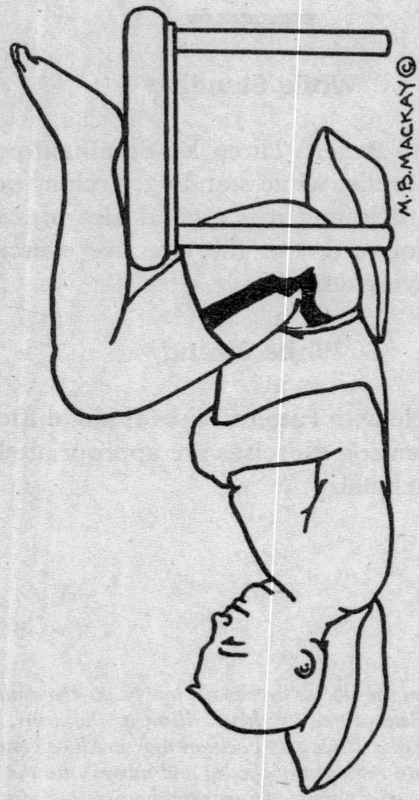
M.B.MACKAY©

While Lying

Position rather than movement is often the pain control exercise for Pattern Three. Simply lying on your stomach may be enough to reduce the typical leg pain. For some, even this position is too much and the best relief is obtained by lying over one or two pillows placed under the pelvis. As symptoms diminish, progress by removing a pillow.

Resting on your elbows, like a child watching television, is more aggressive. Concentrate on letting your lower back sag and monitor your typical leg pain as a measure of success. The sloppy push-up described for Pattern One becomes worthwhile as symptoms subside, but rather than repeating the movement, hold the extended position for a few seconds. The usefulness of the exercise is measured by the reduction or upward migration of the leg pain as it centralizes to the middle of the low back.

Oddly, some people find relief from Pattern One pain in the opposite position, lying on their

Leg pain relief in Pattern Three can result from lying with the knees above the stomach. Cushion the head and buttocks with small pillows and rest the calves on a chair seat or stool. As a rule, the tighter the tuck the less pain in the leg.

backs with their knees bent and their calves resting on the seat of a chair. Flex the hips enough to put the knees above the abdomen. For added comfort, tuck one pillow under the buttocks and another under the head. If both the flexed and extended positions work, alternate them to remain pain free.

PATTERN FOUR —BACK

While Standing

Control of the typical leg symptoms consistent with pattern Four requires changing both your standing and walking posture. The basis of all the exercises is the "pelvic tilt". Start by standing against a flat surface and move your feet forward two or three inches. Press the small of your back against the wall by tightening your buttocks and rolling up the front of your pelvis Feel your stomach draw in and your chest lift. Repeat this movement until it becomes automatic then try and hold the posture as you step away from the wall. Maintaining the pelvic tilt while walking is a challenge.

Many people find it easier to practice this exercise while lying on their backs. When they master the position they can translate it to a standing posture.

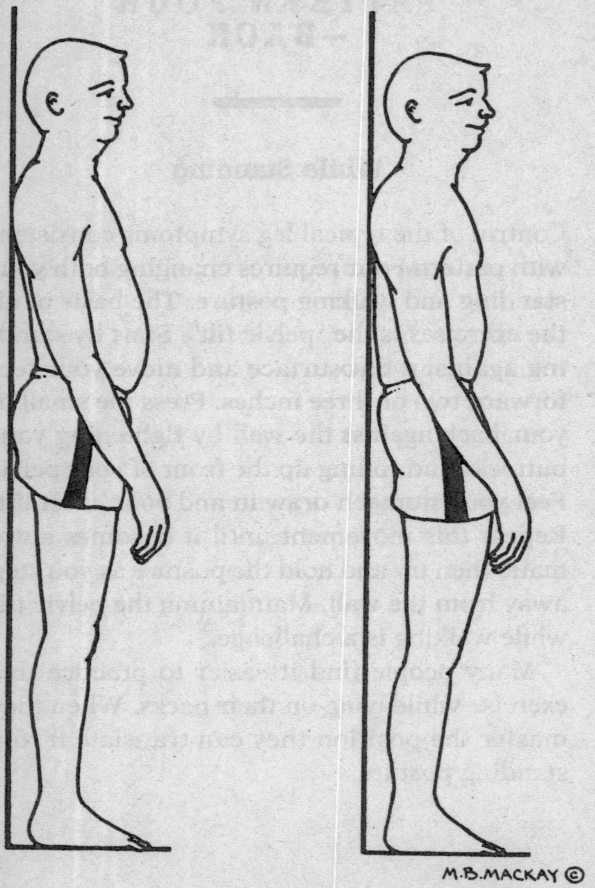
M.B.MACKAY ©

While Sitting

Pain control exercises for Pattern Four are the same as those for Pattern Two.

While Lying

Lying on your back with your knees bent, flatten your lower back against the floor by rolling your pelvis up. Tighten your buttocks but keep them down and don't lift your feet. You will feel the effect in your abdomen and your lumbar spine.

Maintaining this pelvic tilt uses the abdominal muscles, so Pattern Four is the only pattern where pain control includes a strengthening component. Use the flexion exercises described in the next section.

It can be difficult to perform a standing pelvic tilt. Pushing the back against a wall helps to identify the correct position. Tighten the abdomen, clench the buttocks and roll the pelvis forward. Hold the tilt and step away from the wall.

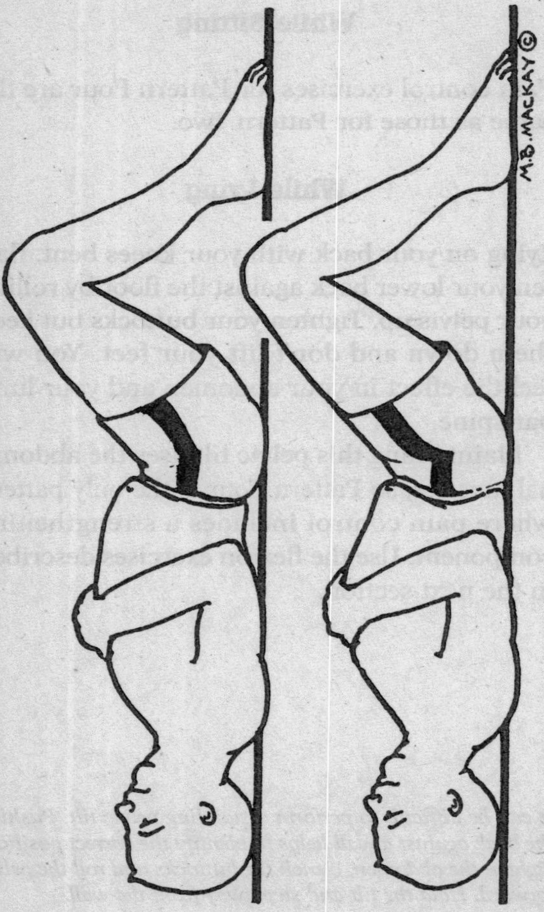
M.B. MACKAY ©

The pelvic tilt is the first step for most abdominal strengthening exercises. Flatten the small of the back by rotating the pelvis and tightening the buttocks. Keep the feet on the floor but don't push with the legs.

YOUR PROGRAM FOR PATTERN FIVE

Posture

Because the primary treatment objective is to prevent pain from dictating activity, change your position frequently following a predetermined schedule—a schedule that has no regard for pain. It is not difficult to identify the limits imposed by Pattern Five. Set goals well within these boundaries. On a good day, meeting your target poses no challenge. On a bad day, even simple tasks may seem impossible, so start at a level you can manage and progress at a pace you can endure. An altered perception of pain does not eliminate the possibility of an underlying mechanical pattern. Temporary control of that physical discomfort is a great place to start.

Patterns One and Three

Standing with one foot up on a step or stool produces an optimal curve in the low back and helps to position the head above the shoulders. Sitting with a lumbar roll has the same benefits. Lying with a cervical roll or towel around your waist to prevent the spine from sagging is almost always helpful. When you assess the value of the night rolls, be sure to distinguish between the inevitable discomfort the rolls initially produce and any alteration in your typical pain.

Lying on your stomach, perhaps resting on your elbows, may reduce your symptoms. For Pattern Three, this position can be alternated with one in which you lie on your back with your knees bent and your calves resting on a bench or the seat of a chair. Details of these positions are found on page 99. Remember to change positions frequently and systematically before your pain forces you to move.

Patterns Two and Four

Bending forward usually produces short-term pain control, but remaining in a flexed posture almost guarantees that the symptoms will return. Establish a routine where flexion is often repeated but never sustained.

While standing, gently lower your chin toward your chest or bend forward to place your hands on your knees. Hold the position for a few moments then straighten up.

As you sit, use your arms to lower your upper body toward your thighs, but don't stay in that position more than a minute or two.

A rolled towel under your neck or at your waist effectively reduces the pain when you lie down. Instructions on the proper use of the cervical and lumbar rolls are on pages 32 and 77.

Because Pattern Four pain is brought on by activity, this pattern poses a particular problem. The substitution you pick to defeat your pain could be the activity that initiated your pain in the first place. Choose carefully. Holding a flexed posture by contracting your stomach muscles while walking, or reducing the arch in the low back with a pelvic tilt are usually the best ways to begin. There is a description of the pelvic tilt on page 101.

While [illegible], gently [illegible] your [illegible] [illegible] and [illegible] hands on your knees. Hold the pose for just a few moments [illegible].

As you sit up, [illegible] toward your [illegible] position more than a [illegible].

A rolled towel under your neck or in your waist [illegible]

[illegible]

Exercises

The specific pain control exercises you select will be based on the mechanical pattern you are experiencing. In Pattern Five, however, the maneuvers themselves are unlikely to provide lasting benefit. Here, as symptoms reflect the heightened perception of pain, the mechanical problem is only a minor factor.

As important as the choice of exercise is the schedule for their use. Plan your program with reference to the time of day or day of the week; choose anything that has no relation to the pain. At first, the exercise will be painful. Schedule as many sessions a day as you can manage but perform only a few repetitions for each exercise. Pay close attention to your technique; it is more important to do the exercise properly than to do it quickly.

When you have set your goals, write them down and be specific. List the time you will start and the time you will stop, the exercises you have chosen and the number of repetitions you intend to perform. Mark a sheet of paper with spaces in which you can indicate successful completion.

Before you begin, plan your progression. Decide how long you will continue before you increase the number of sessions per day or the number or repetitions per exercise. This determination should have nothing to do with pain although pain will certainly try to interfere. Start slowly and move forward steadily. Failing at an overly ambitious attempt will reinforce the sense of futility commonly associated with Pattern Five. Measured progress is the right idea.

The goals you set are a unique reflection of your situation. One man found his back pain so severe that he was only able to walk to the house next door before being forced home. His first target was to walk to that house five times a day. His progression was to increase his walking distance to the next house on the block and then to the house after that. His record of accomplishment was measured in houses and for him it worked.

Chart your activities meticulously. A list of three days' exercise may not seem significant but a visual record of three months' progress can have a profound positive effect.

Pattern One

Pain control exercises in Pattern One are generally repeated retractions for the neck and frequent arching backward for the lumbar spine. Many patients begin the exercise program lying down to reduce the effect of gravity.

Progression includes additional exercises or increased repetitions. It can be as simple as moving the same program from a recumbent to an upright position. Lay out the steps in your progression then make it happen regardless of fluctuations in the level of pain.

Details of the pain control exercises for Pattern One in the neck are found on pages 35-39. Pain control for Pattern One in the low back is described on pages 85-87.

Pattern Two

Bending forward, the standard pain control maneuver for Pattern Two, can be difficult due to the intensity of the pain but, particularly in Pattern Five, hurt is not harm.

Start in a seated position and use your arms to raise and lower your upper body over your thighs. Progress to standing and finally to lying down. Move slowly and stay under control. Flexion exercises for the neck are described on pages 47-51. Routines for low back flexion are found on pages 138-149.

Pattern Three

The infrequent occurrence and relatively short duration of this pattern make its combination with Pattern Five unusual. Because Pattern Three is the most dramatic and feared of the mechanical patterns, however, it is frequently cited by the Pattern Five patient as the unrecognized source of the unremitting pain.

Arm or leg dominant symptoms usually respond to exercises done lying down. Treatment for Pattern Three in the neck is described on pages 49-51. Management of Pattern Three involving the low back is discussed on pages 97-99.

Pattern Four

The abdominal strengthening exercise described

on page 101, is the best place to begin. Reducing the curve of the low back requires conscious effort and muscular control. Strengthening exercises take time to produce effect, and in Pattern Five the effort is always painful. Prepare a realistic and achievable routine and stay with it. It's easy to become discouraged, so review your record of accomplishment frequently.

Because Pattern Five generally appears after prolonged periods of inactivity, all attempts to re-establish movement will hurt. Because the mechanical patterns are rarely well defined and are of secondary importance, the specific exercise selection is sometimes arbitrary. Experiment with a variety of approaches, times and repetitions. Develop any routine that gives you the greatest pain control. There is no risk; try whatever you want—but try.

YOUR PROGRAM FOR PROTECTION

Pain control maneuvers need to be repeated frequently and spaced throughout the day. Exercises that reduce the risk of recurrence are best done at regular times and in a designated location away from all unwanted distractions. Start as soon as pain control is established and the acute episode is over.

The program can be brief but it requires effort and commitment. Three half-hour sessions per week is adequate. To add interest divide the complete program into a rotating sequence of different routines.

Choose a series of exercises that suits your personal needs. If your pain remains under control you don't have to progress to the next level of difficulty. Ten repetitions is average but use as few or as many as you need. Begin slowly and allow yourself time to cool down. Stretch before you strengthen and stretch again before you finish. Consider the exercise period your private time. An exercise partner can keep you motivated but you don't need an audience.

POSTURE

The simplest protection is to continue the same posture that relieved your pain. The extreme positions necessary during an acute episode are no longer required and now pain control becomes synonymous with comfort. Balance your head above your shoulders and maintain a relaxed curve in your neck and low back. When standing, place one foot on a step and change position frequently. When sitting, always use a lumbar support and avoid soft, sagging furniture. Keep night rolls of the proper thickness for your neck and low back and use them whenever sleep is disturbed by your typical pain.

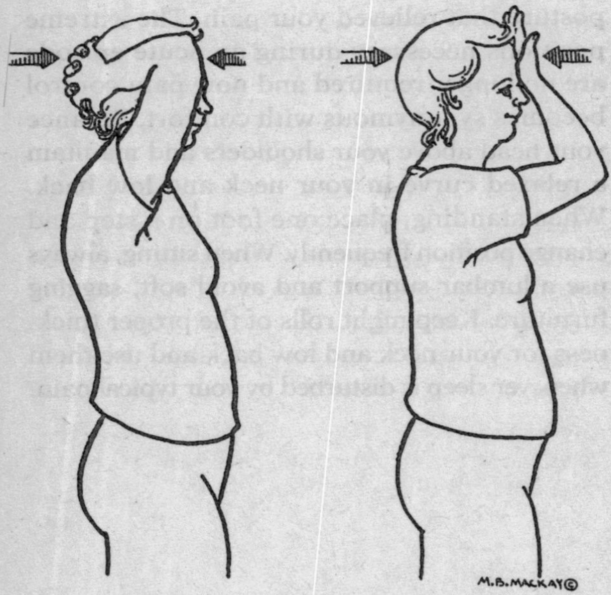
M.B.MACKAY©

EXERCISES FOR THE NECK

Exercises for the neck include exercises that strengthen the muscles of the shoulder girdle.

Exercise 1: Resisted Retraction

With your fingers laced together put your hands behind your head. Push back with your head as you pull forward with your arms. Develop tension but don't move. This type of exercise is called "isometric" which means no distance is travelled; this is a fancy way of saying "stay completely still". If the pressure is too great and you begin to quiver the exercise loses its value and you may resurrect your pain.

Resisted retraction *and* protraction *are isometric exercises. Strength is produced without movement by the action of one muscle group against another. Generate as much force as possible but remain perfectly still.*

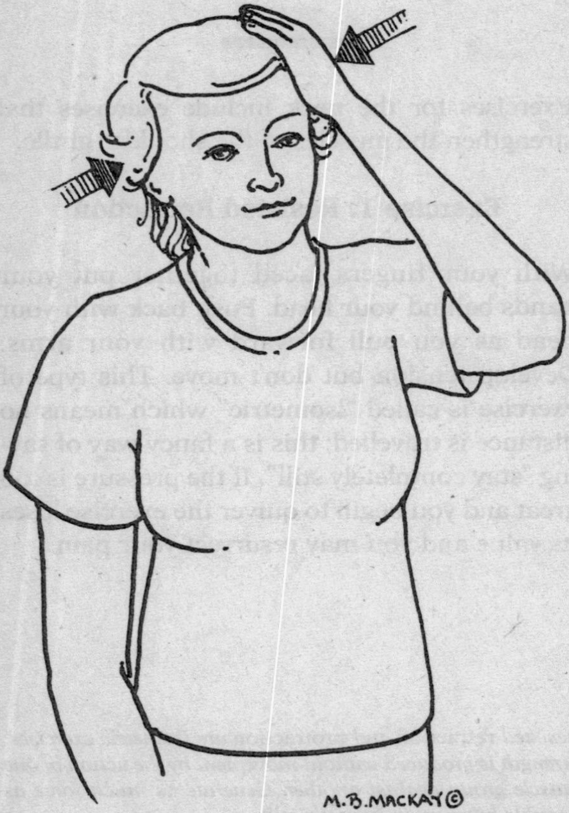
M.B.MACKAY©

Exercise 2: Resisted Protraction

This is similar to Exercise 1 but is performed as you thrust your head forward against resistance. Point your fingers up and press the palms of your hands against your forehead. Note that this is another isometric exercise; don't move.

Exercise 3: Resisted Side Flexion

With the palm of your hand firmly against the side of your head, just above your ear, try to tip your head sideways. Yes, one more isometric exercise. Repeat the same maneuver trying to tip to the other side.

Resisted side flexion *strengthens muscles running diagonally across the neck. Like all isometric exercises, force should be generated without movement.*

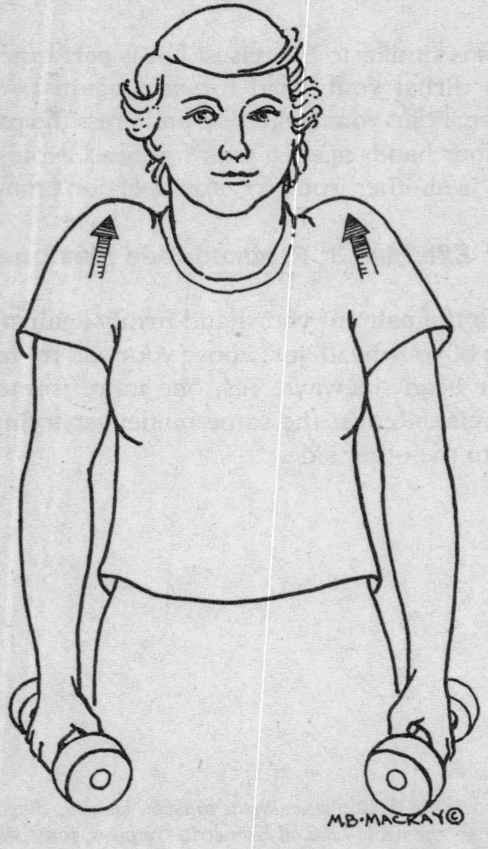
M.B.MACKAY©

Exercise 4: Shoulder Shrugs

With your arms hanging at your sides raise your shoulders toward your ears. The effort uses muscles that suspend your collar bones and shoulder blades—muscles needed for good neck and shoulder posture. Keep your head well balanced so that a line drawn through your ear would pass through the middle of your shoulder. To develop more strength perform the shoulder shrugs holding weights in your hands.

Shoulder shrugs strengthen muscles supporting the arms and stabilizing the neck. Limit movement to the shoulders; avoid moving the head. Perfect the technique before increasing the weight.

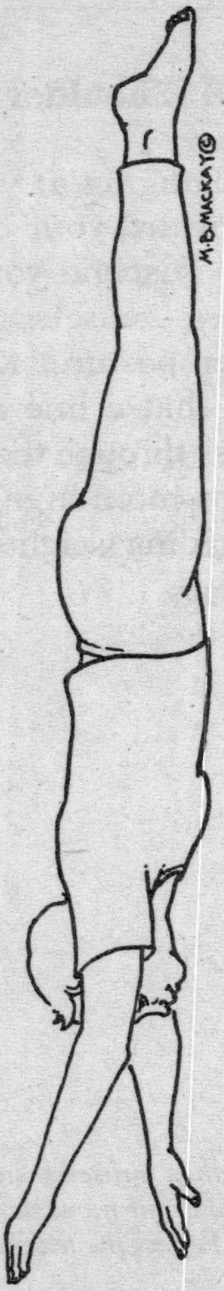
M.B.MACKAY©

EXERCISES FOR THE BACK

EXTENSION

Exercise 1: One Arm Extension

Lie face down with both arms straight out above your head. Raise one hand up six inches above the floor and hold it there. Slowly lower your arm; don't let it fall. Switch to the other side. To increase the difficulty lift both arms together; make the "One Arm Extension" into a "Two Arm Extension".

Prone single arm extension is an easy way to begin strengthening the back muscles. Lifting the arm exercises trunk muscles that steady the spine. Lifting both arms at once requires more trunk strength.

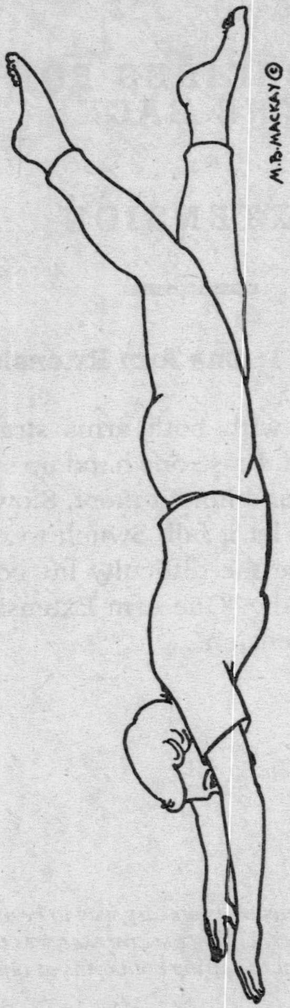
M.B.MACKAY ©

Exercise 2: One Leg Extension

Lie on your stomach. Bend one knee enough to raise your foot and take strain off the low back. Now lift your thigh clear of the floor and hold. Let it down slowly and repeat with the other leg. You can increase the effort of your low back and buttock muscles by keeping your knee straight.

A prone single leg extension requires the back muscles to anchor the spine. Stabilizing the back and pelvis against the weight of the leg requires more strength than working against the weight of one arm.

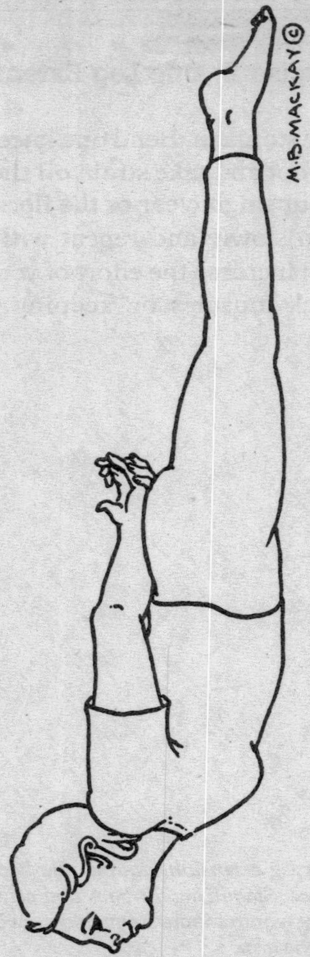
M.B. MACKAY ©

Exercise 3: Trunk Extension

Lie on your stomach and tuck your chin into your chest. Arch your back to raise your head and shoulders. Come up slowly, hold, and relax. This exercise is easiest with your hands resting on your buttocks. It becomes more difficult if you place your hands by your ears and hold your elbows out. The most difficult position is with your arms extended over your head.

Trunk extension elevates the head and shoulders, which strengthens muscles all along the spine. Don't arch the neck. The easiest way to perform this exercise is with the hands behind the back.

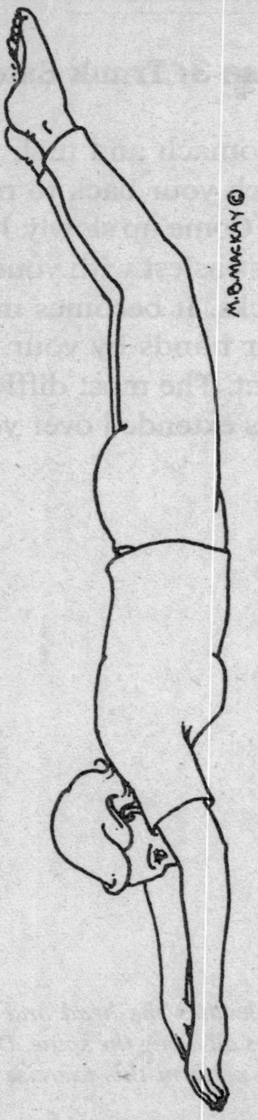
M.B.MACKAY ©

Exercise 4: Double Leg Extension

Lie face down with both knees slightly bent and raise your thighs an inch or two off the floor. Press down with your hands as you lift your legs. Make this exercise more difficult by keeping your legs straight.

The low back strength required for a prone double leg lift is considerably greater than that needed to lift one leg alone. With both legs in the air, the paraspinal muscles are the only source of spinal stability. Balance the upper body by extending the arms above the head.

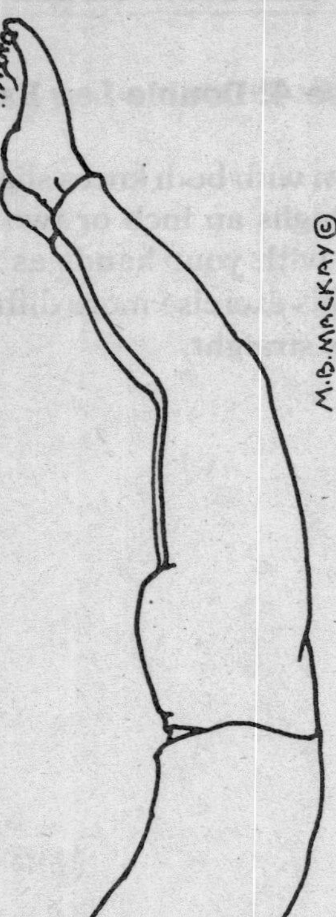
M.B. MACKAY ©

Exercise 5: Trunk and Leg Extension

Lie on your stomach, keep your chin tucked and your knees slightly bent. Raise your head and shoulders and lift your thighs off the floor at the same time. Stay under control; move slowly. The difficulty can be adjusted by changing your arm positions as described for Exercise 3.

Active prone extension *strengthens the back muscles, but holding this position may be uncomfortable forsomeone with Pattern Two back pain. Extend slowly and maintain control. Sudden backward rocking has little value. Hands behind the neck is the position for intermediate difficulty.*

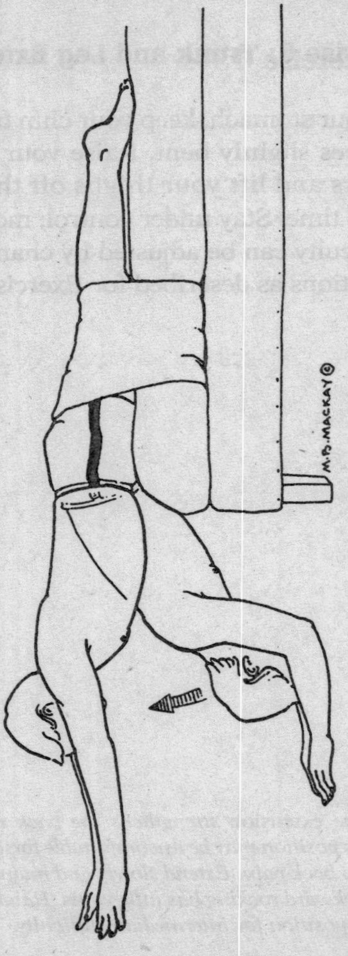
M.D.MACKAY©

Exercise 6: The Horizontal Lift

Hang face down over the edge of a platform or bed. Whether you have an exercise partner or use a belt, be sure that your legs are held securely. Slowly raise yourself to the horizontal position, and then sink back slowly. Keep your chin tucked and don't arch your spine. Modify the difficulty by changing the arm positions as described for Exercise 3.

The horizontal lift is achieved through extension over the edge of a couch, which strengthens the back muscles with arching the back. It is the most efficient extension strengthening exercise. Be sure that the hips and thighs are well secured. Extending the arms above the head is the most difficult variation.

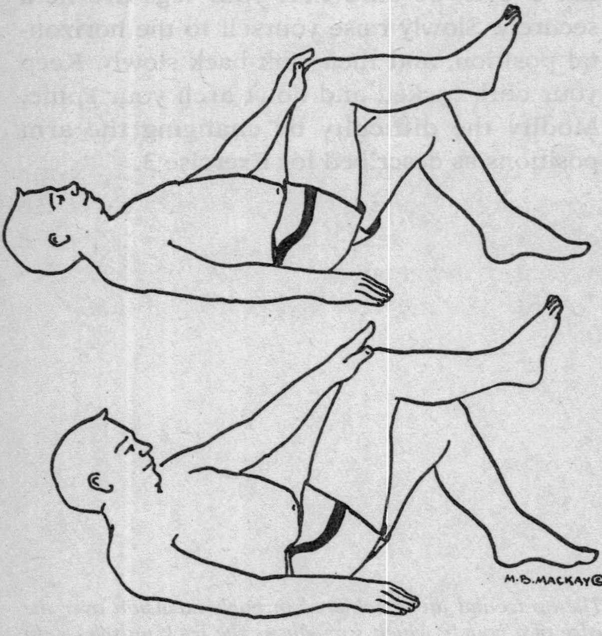
M.B.MACKAY©

EXERCISES FOR THE BACK

FLEXION

Exercise 7: Cross-Arm Knee Push

Lying on your back, place your hand firmly on the opposite knee and push. Hold a pelvic tilt and keep your head back. This is an isometric exercise; one group of muscles works against another and there should be no movement.

The cross-arm knee push is an isometric exercise and acts by tensing the abdominal muscles. The difficulty increases with raising the head and shoulders while maintaining pressure on the knee.

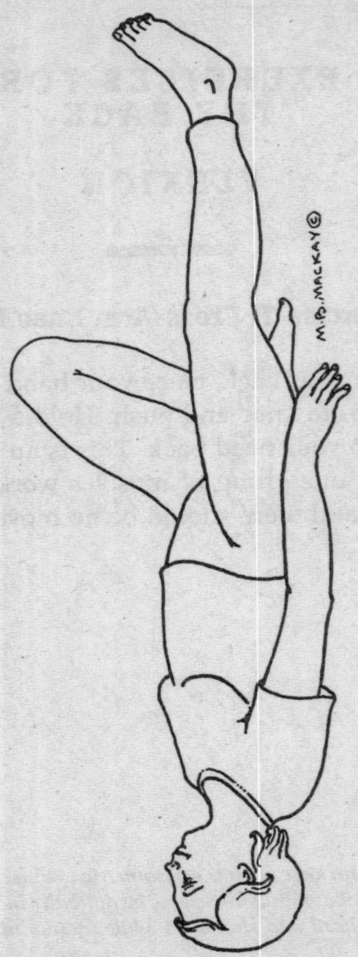
M.D. MACKAY ©

Exercise 8: Single Leg Lift

As you lie on your back, bend one hip and knee and place your foot beside your buttock. This establishes a pelvic tilt. Lift your other leg eight to ten inches above the floor. Keep your knee straight and don't arch your back. Hold for a short count and relax. Perform a number of repetitions before changing legs.

The exercise is easier if you lift your leg with your knee slightly bent. For a more difficult version lift both legs together; make the "Single Leg Lift" into a "Double Leg Lift". With both legs up, keeping your low back flat on the floor requires strong trunk muscles.

A supine single leg lift strengthens the abdominal muscles. Flexing the opposite leg stabilizes the pelvis and prevents an undesirable arch in the low back.

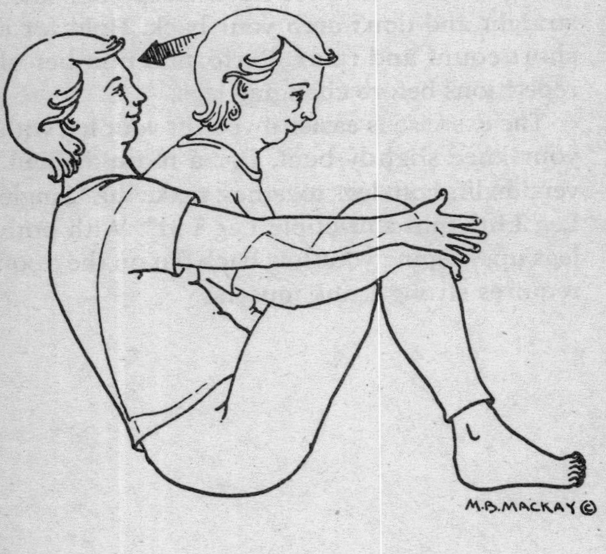
M.B.MACKAY ©

Exercise 9: The Sit Down

Here is one type of Sit-Up that requires very little abdominal strength. Sit on the floor and hug your knees. Lean back slowly without letting go of your legs. When you have gone back as far as your arms will let you, pull yourself up again.

With practice you can transfer control from your arms to your abdomen. Begin by letting go and allowing your upper body to sink to the floor. The slower your descent the more you exercise your stomach.

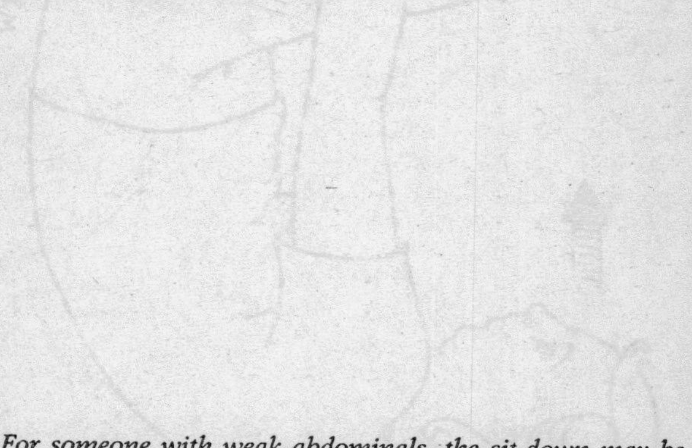

For someone with weak abdominals, the sit-down may be the best way to begin. Grasp the knees and slowly lean backward then use the stomach muscles to return to the starting point. As the span increases, the sit-down becomes a sit-up.

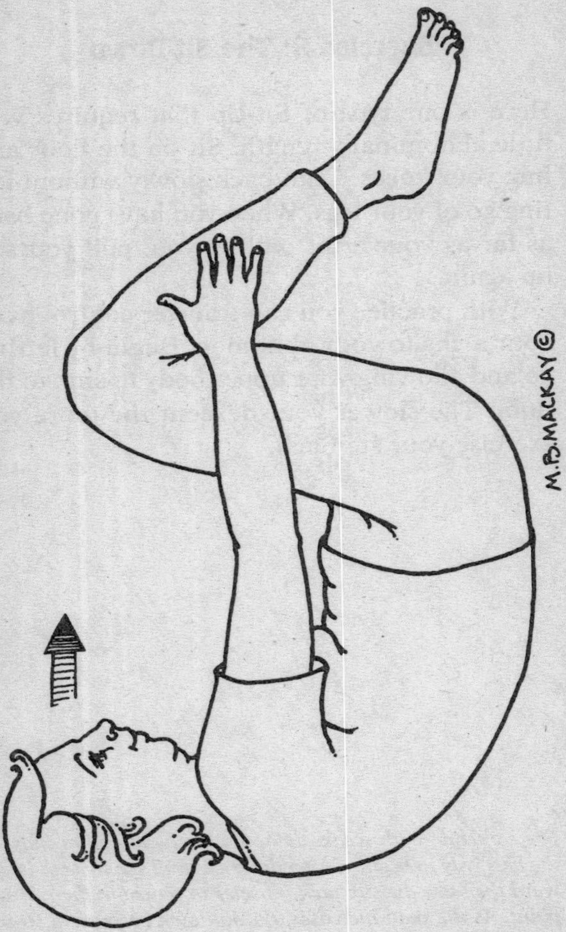
M.B.MACKAY ©

Exercise 10: The Crunch

Lying on your back with both knees bent, raise your head and shoulders and your legs at the same time. As you try to touch your knees to your forehead remember it is the movement, not the contact, that matters. Rocking back and forth to use your body's momentum defeats the purpose. Move slowly to maintain control.

The easiest way to do this exercise is with the arms extended alongside the knees. The intermediate position has the arms folded across the chest. For the most difficult variation hold the elbows out and place the hands over the ears.

The crunch brings the knees up and the shoulders forward at the same time. Keep the movement controlled and avoid flexing the neck. Holding the arms straight out in front is the easiest position for a flexion exercise.

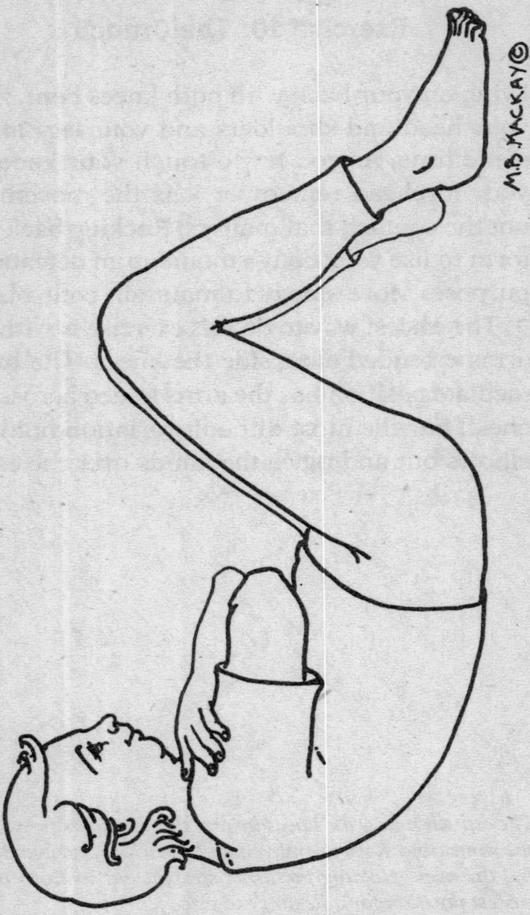
M.B. MACKAY©

Exercise 11: The Sit-Up

The first part of the Sit-Up, raising your trunk until your shoulder blades clear the floor, is the hardest and most valuable. Lift your upper body in one piece with your chin tucked and your head back. Keep your knees bent. Your feet should be unconstrained and should stay on the floor. Using something to hold the feet down shifts the action away from the abdomen to the hip muscles. Sit up slowly and maintain a pelvic tilt.

The Sit-Up can be made more or less difficult by altering the position of the arms as described for Exercise 10.

Flexing the knees and keeping the feet down during the part sit-up activates the abdominal muscles. Hold a pelvic tilt and elevate the upper body until the shoulder blades clear the floor. Arms crossed over the chest is the position of intermediate difficulty.

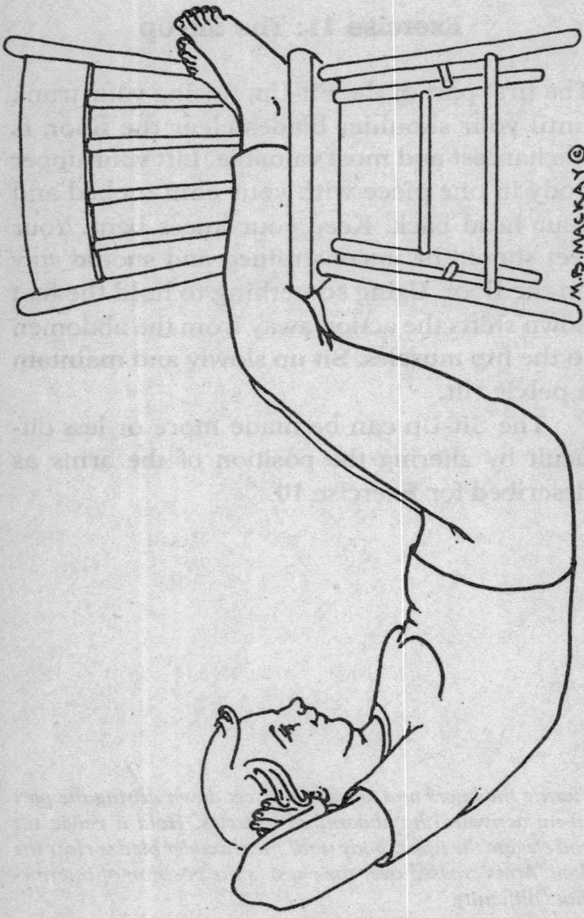
M.D. MACKAY ©

Exercise 12: The Tougher Sit-Up

Bending your hips and knees and resting your calves on a seat prevents your hip flexor muscles from participating and places the entire burden on your abdominal muscles. Keep your head back and your chin down. Raise your shoulders until your shoulder blades clear the floor. This tough Sit-Up can be made tougher by altering the location of your arms as described for Exercise 10.

This is the most difficult sit-up. Resting the legs on a chair eliminates the effect of the hip flexors, and the stomach muscles must do all the work. The most demanding position is with the hands beside the head.

YOUR FINAL INSTRUCTIONS

Most of us will experience neck or back pain, and most of that discomfort will be the result of natural aging within the discs and joints of the spine. You can't stop growing older but you can overcome many of its unpleasant effects through proper posture, frequent pain-control exercise and a program of long-term prevention.

Begin by correcting your posture. Your goal is to centralize, reduce or abolish your typical pain and the posture that delivers these results is the right one for you. It may seem extreme or uncomfortable but you can't harm your back with good posture.

Once you have a pain-control routine that works, use it often. The more opportunities you give your neck or low back to rest and recover, the more rapidly they will reward you by becoming pain free. You may feel self-conscious about performing some of these exercises but the choice is yours and it's clear; live with the occasional curious stare or live with the pain.

Don't confuse maneuvers for rapid pain control with exercises to reduce the threat of further attacks. Protection is achieved through continuous posture modification and increasing muscular endurance. It takes time and effort. Most people achieve a balanced program combining flexion and extension to strengthen the muscles of the abdomen and those that surround the trunk. The task can be arduous, but it should never re-create the pain from which you have just escaped.